Relationship Between Healthcare Delivery, Public Policy, and Public and Community Health

Cognella Series on
Public and Community Health Nursing

Relationship Between Healthcare Delivery, Public Policy, and Public and Community Health

Anita Finkelman, MSN, RN

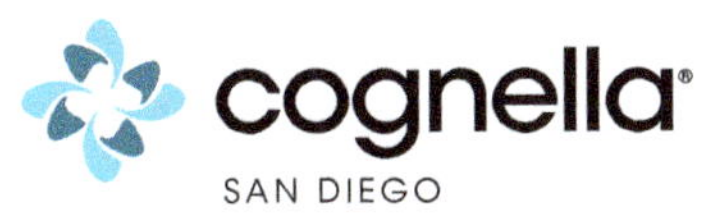

Bassim Hamadeh, CEO and Publisher
Amanda Martin, Publisher
Amy Smith, Senior Project Editor
Rachel Kahn, Production Editor
Jess Estrella, Senior Graphic Designer
Kylie Bartolome, Licensing Specialist
Natalie Piccotti, Director of Marketing
Kassie Graves, Senior Vice President, Editorial

Printed in the United States of America.

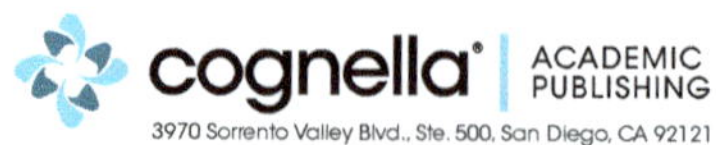

This project is dedicated to all the students who have taught me during my years of professional practice in clinical and academic settings. I also recognize the nurses who have provided care daily during the difficult time of a pandemic, treating all equally in all settings and communities, and hold special thoughts for those nurses who experienced illness and lost their lives as they worked to improve the health of their communities.

Contents

ACTIVE LEARNING

This book has interactive activities available to complement your reading.

Your instructor may have customized the selection of activities available for your unique course. Please check with your professor to verify whether your class will access this content through the Cognella Active Learning portal (http://active.cognella.com) or through your home learning management system.

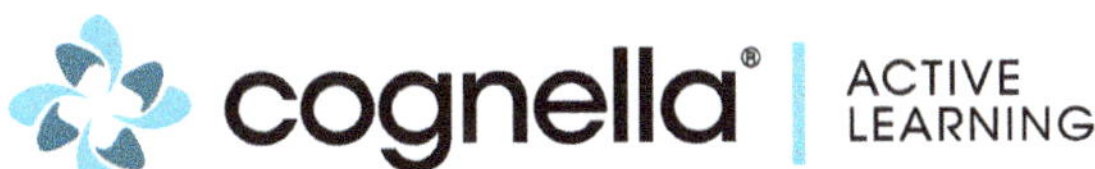

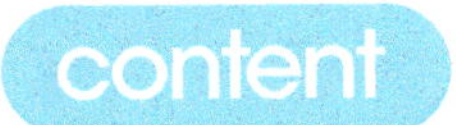

Preface

Effective healthcare delivery requires teams and teamwork in all types of settings, including public and community health services. Designed to support current standards and goals for health care, *Relationship Between Healthcare Delivery, Public Policy, and Public and Community Health* provides an examination of public health policy and its implications for public and community health services. This content focuses on an examination of the policy development process including the legislative process. Public and private health policies are complex and affect services, professional practice, and the healthcare workforce. This process requires engagement from many stakeholders, individual healthcare providers and organizations, and must include input from health profession education, communities and government (local, state, and federal), insurers, those involved in health policy and health research, and consumers. As is true for all types of healthcare services, policy development must consider diversity, equity, and inclusion; the social determinants of health; disparities; population health; and vulnerable populations.

Acknowledgments

I thank my family for their support of my writing and professional endeavors over many years: Fred, Shoshannah, and Deborah—and especially my grandson, Matanel Yizhar, who teaches me daily that learning is constant as well as caring. Thank you to Amanda Martin, a long-time publishing colleague who reached out to me to connect again to develop this project. The Cognella team cannot be praised enough for their professionalism and creativity: Amy Smith for directing editing guidance and keeping me on track; Rachel Kahn for her production leadership; Dani Grandsher, Haley Brown, and all the others who helped with the development of methods supporting creative student engagement in learning and effective faculty resources; Jeannine Rees for guiding production; Natalie Piccotti, who leads the marketing initiative; and so many others who have helped on this project behind the scenes.

Relationship Between Healthcare Delivery, Public Policy, and Public and Community Health

Learning Outcomes

1. Examine the relationship between healthcare delivery, public policy, and public and community health.
2. Compare public and private policy.
3. Analyze the need to integrate equity and other related factors in public and community health policy.
4. Describe the development of policies and relevance of the legislative process to public policy and health care.
5. Examine the impact of funding and reimbursement on public and community health policy.
6. Discuss the importance of research and evidence-based practice supporting public policy.
7. Examine current issues and relationship to public and community health policy.
8. Formulate a summary statement highlighting key points about the relationship among healthcare delivery, public policy, and public and community health.

Key Terms

Advocacy
Artificial intelligence (AI)
Biosurveillance
Coalition
Community
Diversity, equity, inclusion, and accessibility (DEIA)
Evidence-based practice (EBP)
Evidence-informed health policy
Health equity
Health literacy
Health in All Policies (HiAP) model
Legislative process
Lobbying
Mitigation
Not-for-profit organizations
Policy brief

Politics
Political action committee (PAC)
Private policy
Public health authority
Public health law
Public policy
Population health
Regulations
Reimbursement
Situational awareness
Social determinants of health (SDOH)
Stakeholders
Triple Aim
STEEEP®
Upstream-midstream-downstream public health model
Vulnerable population

Introduction

Policies are crucial elements in understanding and ensuring public and community health. This content examines these policies and how they are developed, implemented, and evaluated. There are many **stakeholders**, or persons and organizations that have a strong interest in public health policy, including public and private stakeholders that need to be engaged in the policymaking process.

Demonstrating one example of the importance of public policy is engagement of the American Public Health Association (APHA) as it recognizes National Public Health Week annually. The title for the 2023 week was Centering and Celebrating Cultures in Health, and the week's focus was on the following:

> Feeling like we belong, being a part of our communities and fostering cultural connections supports our health and the quality of our lives. We want everyone to know they can make their communities healthier, safer and stronger when we support and stay engaged with one another ... focusing not just on what we can do as individuals, but what we can do as communities to protect, prioritize, and influence the future of public health. (APHA, 2023a)

Demonstrating the importance of policies and stakeholder engagement, the APHA calls for action with the following activities and provides resources and support for stakeholders to engage in these actions and the policy process to improve public health (APHA, 2023b):

- Contact members of Congress to urge them to support public health funding in the fiscal year (FY) 2024 appropriations process.
- Contact members of Congress to urge them to support legislation to prevent gun violence.

- Contact members of Congress to urge them to protect public health from the impacts of climate change.
- Oppose cuts to critical public health programs in debt limit negotiations.

The following content examines the process, activities, stakeholders, and other relevant issues in policymaking. The APHA is an example of a **not-for-profit organization** that represents public and community health organizations and providers and is involved in policymaking. The U.S. Congress is mentioned in these activities, and government is critical in policymaking, as discussed in this content. There are many methods used to improve and support policy with varied stakeholders, as discussed later, such as government agencies, government (local, state, and federal), and the private sector, such as healthcare professionals and organizations, as well as the development of many resources that guide policy, such as the National Healthcare Quality and Disparities Report (NHQDR) and Healthy People 2030.

Public and Private Policy: Implications for Public and Community Health

Public health policies are not simple and affect many people, with the recognition that some problems require a group or community effort. Public health departments in local communities and states need to respond to complex problems. Many of the problems addressed by public and private health policies may lead to response options that may be challenged and not accepted by some in the community or influential stakeholders (Interlandi, 2020). For example, during the COVID-19 pandemic, some public health interventions were criticized. Some people refused to follow the public health recommendations such as using masks, complained about difficulties with safety measures used in public transportation, disagreed with policy to track quarantine viewing this as a privacy issue, and so on. Politicians may be involved, as they were with the pandemic. This aggravated the response from many sectors. Some politicians, government staff, experts, and consumers questioned the motivation of government and politicians and refused to accept policies that were designed to protect the public. This public health crisis experience emphasizes the need for better policies, an improved policymaking process that includes the implementation and evaluation of policies, and a serious examination of routine health policymaking and preparing for future public health emergency needs. Public health communication is also a critical element that requires consideration in sharing health policies with the public and with healthcare providers and organizations to avoid misinformation and conflicts.

Public and private policy are developed and implemented by different sources and affect different aspects of public and community health, although some have impact on the same healthcare services. The following content discusses **public policy** and its implications and its relationship to **private policies.**

Public Health

Prior to examining policy and public and community health, it is important to understand public health. The main goal of public health is to promote and protect the health of people and the communities where they live, learn, work, and play. Countries that focus on public health recognize that these services are integral and important to the country's health and the healthcare delivery system. These countries typically have more effective data sharing as their health delivery system is viewed as one system rather than having a sharp line between acute and public health care. The United States has the latter system, and this has an impact on the public health perspective and weakened public health effectiveness. "A public health person in charge of a district, state, or country is very clear about who is included in the population they serve. Health care [acute care], on the other hand, for the most part sees the people who come through the doors as their population" (Twum-Danso, 2022). It is important to ensure that these two perspectives of health care are combined (collaborate and coordinate), or there will be gaps in services that have a negative impact on health outcomes. This type of healthcare system and view of health requires clear policies supporting the goals and activities.

Public health is viewed from different perspectives

> whether called partnership, collaboration, or cross-sectoral engagement, working with a diverse range of actors across multiple settings is considered core practice and a logical means to address the many determinants of health that lie outside the reach of public health systems. These relationships take many forms, including public–private partnerships, nonprofit–private partnerships, and public–nonprofit partnerships ... or cross-sector partnerships while maintaining clear distinctions between the public, nonprofit, and private sectors. (Johnston & Finegood, 2015, p. 255)

Policymaking must consider all these factors when public health policy is required. Given the size and variation in the United States, communities may have various requirements due to their demographics, location, and economics, but they all should plan for and support healthy living environments with services to support their community's health, preventing illness when possible and supporting wellness. Acute care is also important, but it differs from public and community health, which is broader in its scope. Private policy focuses more on acute care, such as policies developed by healthcare clinical organizations and professional organizations. Rather than just focusing on illness and treatment, communities need to examine many factors that affect the health and wellness of children and adults of all ages. For example, to maintain the health of individuals, families, and populations, communities (local, state, and national) need to ensure effective access to:

- Healthy and safe housing and living environment
- Safe water and nutrition
- Education
- Employment
- Safe and accessible transportation to go to work, school, and meet other needs
- Parks and exercise for children and adults
- Safe environment, controlling crime, violence, and drug use
- Social activities for all ages
- Health care and prevention for physical and mental health needs for individuals, families, and populations that are accessible and high-quality
- Occupational health (health and safety)
- Government support of public health

Other examples of public health concerns include providing safety on roads; ensuring the use of seatbelts and automobile child restraints; reducing the use of drugs and alcohol; maintaining smoke-free indoor environments; implementing school nutrition programs; providing access to school nurses; providing immunization access for children and adults; ensuring accessible, safe water; providing effective emergency response resources for health needs and during weather and other related emergencies, including public alerts; and maintaining safety during fires and floods. Public and community health also requires management support, which involves collecting data and tracking diseases and injuries, providing public health information to all in the community, collaborating with all types of healthcare providers, and supporting local and state academic healthcare profession education institutions and research. To meet all of their needs and services, communities require funding and effective management of public health budgets, which is discussed later in the content. Support from many types of public health staff must be considered to ensure an effective public health workforce, including public health administrators, health educators, first responders, health inspectors (i.e., in restaurants, businesses), researchers and technologists for data collection and analysis, public health information specialists who share information with the public, elected officials and staff, and healthcare professionals, social workers, sanitation experts and staff, nutritionists, epidemiologists, community planners, occupational health safety experts, and public and community health nurses.

Public and community health should support the 10 essential public health services. See **Appendix A** for a description of these services, which are influenced by public and private policies. Along with these critical services, the APHA has developed a national initiative, called Generation Public Health, focused on:

> people, communities and organizations working to ensure conditions where everyone has the opportunity to be healthy. Our vision is to create the healthiest nation in one generation. Change can only happen if we make healthy choices as a society. This means improving everything that impacts health — from housing, education and income to community design, transportation, and our environment. Together, we can all be the generation that changes the course of health in America. (APHA, 2022)

This initiative emphasizes that everyone has a right to good health.

The Health Resources and Services Administration (HRSA), a U.S. Department of Health and Human Services (HHS) agency, mission and strategic plan goals support the need for public policy "to improve health outcomes and achieve health equity through access to quality services, a skilled health workforce, and innovative, high-value programs" (HRSA, 2023a). One of its goals is to take actionable steps to meet the mission, and this requires policy making related to many aspects of public health such as development of community partnerships, supporting development of the healthcare workforce (funding for education and other workforce needs), and improving access to services, such as prevention as guided by resources provided by the Office of Disease Prevention and Health Promotion (ODPHP), which is part of HHS. The ODPHP also manages the Healthy People 2030 initiative, which is a public health initiative that is based on critical health policy to maintain a healthy nation (ODPHP,

2021). **Appendix B** provides more information on Healthy People. It was established by a 1979 policy decision made by the U.S. Surgeon General. "Laws and policies are critical determinants of health and well-being. They encourage positive behaviors and discourage harmful behaviors, and they can enhance or worsen health, health equity, health disparities, and health literacy. Recognizing their contribution to conditions in the environments in which people are born, live, learn, work, play, worship, and age, and people's experiences of these conditions, the HHS considered the roles of law and policy throughout its development of Healthy People 2030" (Teitelbaum et al., 2021, p. S265).

Public and Private Policies

A **public policy** is a course of action (e.g., a law, a regulation, a procedure, an administrative action, or an incentive that affects the entire population or a segment of it). It is applied by the government and its services and programs, and it may also need to be applied by private healthcare organizations. Public policies are influenced by individual consumers, healthcare providers and organizations, healthcare professional organizations, and government and politics. A **public health law** is a statute, an ordinance, or a code that focuses on health care and is integrated in public policy. Politics and legislation are processes that assist in the development, implementation, maintenance, and review of policies, as described in later content. Public policies may assist in establishing programs that need to be provided to citizens, whether at the local, state, or federal level, and may provide guidance related to effectiveness or policy outcomes. Public policies are critical to the structure and functions of communities. A **community** is "any configuration of individuals, families, and groups whose values, characteristics, interests, geography, and/or social relations unite them in some way" (National Academy of Medicine [NAM], 2017).

Organization policies are often referred to as ***private policies***. These policies direct an organization by clarifying its structure and guiding its functions to meet its goals. Private policies must consider relevant public policies; for example, when a community clinic develops its policies, the clinic management and staff need to consider the Centers for Medicare & Medicaid Services (CMS) federal and state policies (public policies) that affect services for patients who receive either Medicare or Medicaid **reimbursement** (payment for services). Another example of a federal government department that has a great influence on private health policy is the Centers for Disease Control and Prevention (CDC), which played a major role during the COVID-19 pandemic, as discussed in later content.

Government and Policymaking

Public policies are associated with government: local, tribal, state, and federal as well as global organizations, such as the World Health Organization (WHO), that also influence public policies in the United States. Local (i.e., town, city, county) and state governments vary depending on their locations, demographics, and economic status, although all have a similar structure with an executive branch, such as a mayor for a city or town and a state governor. Local governments have a legislative component that focuses on rules and laws for that local community; however, these laws cannot conflict with state and federal legislation. State governments work closely with their local communities and their governments within their state. There are elected officials and nonelected staff within all levels of government.

The U.S. government is based on federalism, which has an impact on policies and how they are developed and implemented. In this model of government powers and policy, assignments are shared between the states and the national government. Federalism has led to problems when public health needs require a consistent, coordinated approach across the nation, and there may be disagreement among the states and with the federal government (Parmet, 2022). The U.S. constitution does not include health or health care as areas in which the federal government has authority. This is left to the states, but this does not mean the federal government should not be active in public health, as described in the following activities. The federal government has long used its right to regulate international and interstate commerce and to tax and spend for the general welfare to support its activities in ensuring the public's health at a national level. As will be discussed in this content, the COVID-19 pandemic is an example of a situation that can lead to public health conflicts between the states and the federal level. Another way this complex issue of collaboration and coordination of policies between the national government and the states is handled is:

> [M]any federal health programs rely on what is commonly known as cooperative federalism. The federal government sets minimum standards and pays much of the costs. In exchange, the states, federal territories and tribal jurisdictions follow federal guidelines, do much of the on-the-groundwork and, at times, set standards that are even more protective of health than those set by the federal government. (Parmet, 2022)

An example of this is the standards and requirements that the CMS establishes for its coverage of healthcare services for certain populations, as is discussed later in this content.

Before discussing how health policy is developed, it is important to describe the structure and function of government, particularly federal government and the governmental components that have an impact on health policy. The HHS is the major federal department concerned with health. Its mission is to "enhance the health and well-being of all Americans, by providing for effective health and human services and by fostering sound, sustained advances in the sciences underlying medicine, public health, and social services" (HHS, 2023a). The structure of this department is complex, with 12 divisions and nine agencies in the U.S. Public Health Service, which provides direct public health medical, health and engineering services to address disease, conduct research, and care for patients in underserved communities across the nation and globally, as well as three human services agencies. These divisions administer a wide variety of health and human services and are engaged in research to improve health and healthcare services. The secretary of HHS is a presidential cabinet position serving as the key health advisor to the president (HHS, 2023a). **Exhibit 1** identifies the missions of the major HHS agencies and offices that relate to health policy and public and community health (HHS, 2023b).

Exhibit 1: U.S. Department of Health and Human Services: Agencies and Offices

- **The Administration for Children and Families** promotes the economic and social well-being of families, children, individuals, and communities through a range of educational and supportive programs in partnership with states, tribes, and community organizations.
- **The Administration for Community Living** increases access to community support and resources for the unique needs of older Americans and people with disabilities.
- **The Administration for Strategic Preparedness and Response** leads the nation's medical and public health preparedness for, response to, and recovery from disasters and public health emergencies.
- **The Agency for Healthcare Research and Quality's** mission is to produce evidence to make health care safer, higher-quality, more accessible, more equitable, and affordable and to work within HHS and other partners to make sure that the health evidence is understood and used.
- **The Agency for Toxic Substances and Disease Registry** prevents exposure to toxic substances and the adverse health effects and diminished quality of life associated with exposure to hazardous substances from waste sites, unplanned releases, and other sources of environmental pollution.

- **The Faith-Based and Neighborhood Partnerships** leads the HHS' efforts to build and support partnerships with faith-based and neighborhood organizations to better serve individuals, families, and communities in need.
- **The Centers for Disease Control and Prevention** protects the nation's public health by providing leadership and direction in the prevention and control of diseases and other preventable conditions and responding to public health emergencies.
- **The Centers for Medicare and Medicaid Services** combines the oversight of the Medicare program, the federal portion of the Medicaid program and state Children's Health Insurance Program, the Health Insurance Marketplace (the Affordable Care Act [ACA] provision), and related quality assessment activities.
- **The Food and Drug Administration** ensures that food is safe, pure, and wholesome; human and animal drugs, biological products, and medical devices are safe and effective; and electronic products that emit radiation are safe.
- **The Health Resources and Services Administration** provides health care to people who are geographically isolated or economically or medically vulnerable and supports healthcare workforce development and supply.
- **The Indian Health Service** provides American Indians and Alaska Natives with comprehensive health services by developing and managing programs to meet their health needs.
- **The National Institutes of Health** supports biomedical and behavioral research in the United States and abroad, conducts research in its own laboratories and clinics, trains researchers, and promotes collecting and sharing medical knowledge to support evidence-base practice.
- **The Office for Civil Rights** ensures that individuals receiving services from HHS-conducted or HHS-funded programs are not subject to unlawful discrimination, individuals and entities can exercise their conscience regarding their rights and religious freedom, and individuals can access and trust the privacy and security of their health information.
- **The Office of Global Affairs** provides leadership and expertise in global health diplomacy to contribute to a safer, healthier world, collaborating globally.
- **The Office of Inspector General** protects the integrity of HHS programs (i.e., regarding ethical and legal concerns) as well as the health and welfare of the program participants.
- **The Office of Intergovernmental and External Affairs** represents both the government and external perspective in federal policymaking and clarifies the federal perspective to government officials and external parties.

- **The Office of Medicare Hearings and Appeals** administers nationwide hearings for the Medicare program to ensure equitable services.
- **The Office of National Security** manages departmentwide programs and provides oversight, policy direction, standards, and performance assessments in the areas of intelligence, counterintelligence, insider threat, cyber threat intelligence, information security, national personnel security, homeland security, and the safeguarding of the nation.
- **The Office of the National Coordinator for Health Information Technology** provides counsel for the development and implementation of a national health information technology (HIT) framework.
- **The Substance Abuse and Mental Health Services Administration**, part of the Public Health Service, improves access and reduces barriers to high-quality, effective programs and services for individuals with substance use and mental disorders as well as for their families and communities.

Source: U.S. Department of Health and Human Services. (2023). Health and human services agencies and offices. *https://www.hhs.gov/about/agencies/hhs-agencies-and-offices/index.html*

An important example of an HHS agency is the CDC, which was established in 1946 as the Communicable Disease Center. At that time, there was a national concern about malaria spreading across the country, which was viewed as a major public emergency. This experience was new for the country. Since the HHS was the important health department in the federal government, a major public health policy decision was made regarding the most appropriate location for this center, which later became known as the *Centers for Disease Control and Prevention*, although it is still referred to as the *CDC*. The agency's activities and services have expanded, and it is now an important resource for state and local health needs, providing support to both state and local health departments. The goal was to establish a U.S. public health service, and these policy decisions served as the framework for the current CDC. Since the CDC's development was driven initially by the need for national infectious disease control, this continues to be a major focus even though many other public health needs and services requiring policies are now recognized and part of HHS and the CDC, including chronic illness, opioid epidemic, violence, weather-related disasters, health problems related to food products, medication shortages, infant formula safety and availability, terrorism, and public health needs for immigrants and refugees. There is also greater attention given to Public Health Emergency Preparedness and

Response (PHEPR) for communicable diseases and public health disasters (e.g., weather-related, terrorism). However, its major activities are collecting and analyzing data it provides guidance to healthcare professionals and organizations and for consumers to ensure that they are healthy. The agency collaborates closely with states and healthcare organizations (acute care and public and community health) to ensure that policies are followed, and information shared.

Several of the HHS agencies mentioned in **Exhibit 1** have significant responsibilities that affect health policy, and their staff work closely with

Exhibit 2: HHS Agencies

- **AHRQ:** This agency is involved in health systems research, practice improvement, and data and analytics. It is responsible for the development of the NHQDR, which affects health policy and public and private decisions through its provision of data and guidance.
- **HRSA:** This agency is involved in ensuring health for many who struggle to gain access to health care when they need it and supports grants and training to ensure the provision of services that include maternal-child health, primary care, HIV/AIDS services, and services for rural communities. The HRSA is also engaged in workforce development with its scholarships and loan repayment programs for healthcare professionals. The HRSA Office of Diversity, Inclusion and Civil Rights is engaged in policy that promotes compliance with federal civil rights laws, supporting inclusive work environments and preventing discrimination in the HRSA's programs and services.
- **CDC:** One of the CDC's major responsibilities is the administration of Healthy People 2030, which requires the collection and assessment of data to determine whether goals and objectives are met, all of which affect health policy, and to provide data and recommendations. A more detailed discussion of the CDC is found in this content due to the agency's critical responsibilities related to ensuring public health.
- **CMS:** CMS policies are significant sources of guidance and reimbursement for public health. Local and state health departments need to be aware of CMS' decisions and their impact on health services and the health of the community.
- **FDA:** This agency addresses needs and evaluates the food and drug supply. As was experienced in 2022 to 2023, there was a shortage of infant formula, and this had an impact on infant nutrition and health. Drug shortages are

discussed later in this content and represent a critical need for policies that can ensure reliable access to and safety of drugs.

- **NIH:** The NIH guides health and science research and includes the National Institute for Nursing Research (NINR), which is concerned with nursing practice and research and the need for effective public health.

healthcare organizations and professionals. **Exhibit 2** discusses some of these agencies and highlights their missions.

In addition to recognizing the federal government's health-related department and agencies, the judicial system also has an impact on policies. For example, state laws may be questioned in the federal court system and the Supreme Court, such as state laws on abortion. Interstate issues also arise, as was experienced during the COVID-19 pandemic when some states wanted to limit residents' travel from other states to their home state. Additionally, problems arose regarding a lack of access to medical supplies, which led to competition to obtain them. In these types of situations, the state, federal court system, and Supreme Court may be involved. This type of state–federal system has increased disagreements among the states and thus within the country. This is of particular concern during times of public health crisis. It is important to recognize that the division between the states and the federal government is not always clear. Funding also affects policies' development and implementation. For example, Medicaid funding is shared between the states and CMS (federal government), which then affects how policies are developed, implemented, and evaluated with differences among states as well as the presence of federal policies, which must be considered.

Critique of the Status of the National Public Health System

Demonstrating the importance of health for the nation, the HHS is the nation's leading science-based, data-driven service department that protects the public's health. As described in **Exhibits 1** and **2**, the HHS has many agencies that provide important services related to public and community health and acute care. Some of its agencies were more involved in policies and response to the pandemic, such as the AHRQ, HRSA, FDA, NIH, and, in particular, the CDC. This department has the largest budget of any federal government department, with a FY 2023 budget of $2.73 trillion that was distributed among its 13 subcomponents (USAspending.gov, 2023). This level of funding indicates that the HHS can have a major impact on policies and outcomes and can provide many services and resources.

The government is also involved in assessing the healthcare system. In 2023, AHRQ Director Robert Otto Valdez expressed concerns about the status of the healthcare system, which affects policies:

> We have lots of work ahead of us as we rebuild our healthcare delivery systems to be more resilient to all types of hazards, such as the biological hazard we faced with COVID-19. But, in many parts of our Nation this spring, we also face natural disasters such as flooding, mudslides, and tornadoes. To respond effectively to these emergencies, we must help our Federal and State partners build robust public health systems. But we must also focus on building resilient local healthcare delivery systems and hospitals that provide the high-quality personal healthcare that the people of this Nation want and expect. (Valdez, 2023)

Valdez emphasized that the country must start rebuilding its healthcare delivery systems immediately, focusing on improving patient safety and workforce well-being in hospitals and nursing homes. The goals of these initiatives must focus on quality and safety and recognize that some citizens are not receiving high-quality care. This type of commentary and analysis from Valdez makes it clear that the United States should not wait for another public health emergency. He indicated that the country currently has a public health emergency—a system that needs improvement in the acute care sector and public health and how they collaborate. The weaknesses in the public health infrastructure and workforce have long been ignored and became worse during the pandemic crisis. This cannot continue, or the country will find that it has deeper healthcare delivery problems and will experience a further decrease in the public's health. Additionally, if there is another epidemic or major disaster, the system will not be able to handle it.

In 2022 and 2023, as the COVID-19 pandemic began to decrease, more attention was given to assessing the United States' response to the pandemic and determining who was responsible for critical response elements (Inglesby & Morrison, 2023). The CDC mission focuses on:

> 24/7 to protect America from health, safety, and security threats, both foreign and in the U.S. Whether diseases start at home or abroad, are chronic or acute, curable or preventable, human error or deliberate attack, CDC fights disease and supports communities and citizens to do the same. The CDC

> increases the health security of our nation. As the nation's health protection agency, CDC saves lives and protects people from health threats. To accomplish our mission, CDC conducts critical science and provides health information that protects our nation against expensive and dangerous health threats, and responds when these arise. (CDC, 2022a)

The assessment of status of healthcare services included a review of the CDC due to its important health functions.

The intense scrutiny of the U.S. healthcare system, brought on by concerns during and after COVID-19, has highlighted many issues; however, the most crucial point is regarding the need for improvement within the public health system. Public policy has an impact on the problems and interventions to improve, and the system critique includes a review by private organizations and the government. This is important as it represents a broad review by multiple stakeholders. It is also important to note that after the pandemic and the development of many policies and changes to meet needs of the public health crisis, the country was stressed and ready to return to "normal." Care must be taken to make thoughtful decisions that improve policy, but what happens to the new policies and changes in policies that existed prior to the pandemic? As assessment information is reviewed and plans are made post-pandemic, the United States also must cope with workforce challenges—a workforce who is tired and, in many locations, lacking staff. There are other challenges that relate to COVID-19 that must be considered in policy development (e.g., new vaccines that helped reduce COVID-19), but their long-term value must be assessed along with how to use the vaccine routinely. Policy will need to be developed and communicated to healthcare providers and the public. Some people who had COVID-19 continue to have health problems, representing an unknown area of health issues and interventions. How does this affect communities and healthcare services, including in regard to costs, as well as personal lives? These factors influence health policies.

The Commonwealth Fund is an example of a private-sector policymaking organization that also assessed the status of public health post-pandemic. It is a private foundation that "promotes a high-performing, equitable health care system that achieves better access, improved quality, and greater efficiency, particularly for society's most vulnerable, including people of color, people with low income, and those who are uninsured" (Commonwealth Fund, 2023). The fund emphasizes the need for the federal government to lead a strong and capable public health system that utilizes the HHS to develop and coordinate public health infrastructure, including data and technology; promotes workforce expansion and education to provide public health staff, including community health workers such as the U.S. Public Health Services Commission Corp., to provide services to state, local, tribal, and territorial areas; promotes the establishment and maintenance of laboratories (e.g., for clinical, data collection and analysis, research); and promotes procurement (i.e., timely and sufficient access of supplies and protective equipment, which was a serious problem during the pandemic). The Commonwealth Fund concluded that there is a need for clear leadership in the national public health system that collaborates with state and local public health leadership. Funding is required to improve at all levels. Policy development and public health initiatives should consider health and equity, as is discussed later in the content. Multiple agencies need to coordinate, communicate, and collaborate and ensure a transparent and accountable public health system (Commonwealth Fund Commission [CFC], 2022a; 2022b). In both public and private assessment of the status of the public health system, the conclusion is the same—the problems are not new but have worsened, and improvement is needed.

Assessment for Improvement

What can be done to address these complex issues regarding health and healthcare delivery? One example is the proposed bill Public Health Infrastructure Saves Lives (PHISLA), which would establish a core Public Health Infrastructure Program at the CDC. This proposal supports federal grants for state, local, and tribal and territorial health departments to ensure they have the tools and resources, workforce, and systems to address existing and emerging health threats and reduce health disparities—supporting effective public health infrastructure. Historically, public health funding has tended to focus on diseases or illnesses, such HIV/AIDs or cardiac issues. However, in using this approach, the public health system has limited its resources to assess and respond to broad public health concerns. It has also restricted its routine consideration of policies that reflect the ongoing public health needs of communities, infrastructure, and funding. This has had a negative impact on public health assessment; preparedness and response; ongoing policy development and support; public health communication; the development of public health professionals and organization competencies; and the support of community partnership development, accountability, and equity. PHISLA is significant legislation, but it has not yet been passed or become law—the key message with this bill is that there is a need for consistent funding to support public health infrastructure. This is an example of how policy can be proposed; however, as noted in the following content, policymaking is complex and may not be successful due to the existence of barriers that crop up throughout the process.

It is possible to track federal legislation, and this is a useful tool for healthcare providers to use as it allows them to keep up to date with policy development. Search for updated information on the U.S. Senate bill titled the Public Health Infrastructure Saves Lives Act, S. 674 (Congress.gov, 2022).

Website: https://www.congress.gov/bill/117th-congress/senate-bill/674

Due to the poor evaluation by public and private stakeholders of the CDC outcomes during the pandemic and concerns about the agency's effectiveness prior to the pandemic, the CDC has begun a major improvement effort of its structure and operations The reviews concluded that the "traditional scientific and communication processes were not adequate to effectively respond to a crisis the size and scope of the COVID-19 pandemic" (U.S. Government Accountability Office [GAO], 2022; Mahr, 2022). These problems are not new, but the pandemic made them worse and, more importantly, brought them into public view. The CDC needs to develop and implement new internal systems, processes, and policies to improve its accountability, collaboration, communication, and timeliness. Changes are needed within the CDC and its collaboration with consumers and stakeholders at all levels of the agency and throughout the local, state, and federal government. Particular concerns emphasize the agency's need to (GAO, 2022):

- Share science and data more quickly
- Translate science into practical policy
- Prioritize public health communications, with a focus on the American public
- Develop a CDC workforce ready to respond to future threats
- Promote partnerships

Response to the reviews has already led to proposed changes in health policy (e.g., related to CDC activities and data during times of public health emergencies and in routinely maintaining public health). **Figure 1** describes the proposed CDC data modernization initiative, representing policy that supports improvement and use of data and guiding public health infrastructure. The initiative will take time to implement and evaluate the outcomes, but it is an important improvement step.

The Center for Strategic & International Studies' Commission on Strengthening America's Health Security assessment report notes that "the United States needs a strong, effective, and more accountable national

ACTIVITIES
If we (CDC and partners) do this ...
SHORT-TERM OUTCOMES
... then we expect these changes to occur ...
INTERMEDIATE OUTCOMES
... which will lead to ...
LONG-TERM OUTCOMES
... our ultimate goals.
COORDINATE PEOPLE AND SYSTEMS
Create interoperable systems: federal, state, local, and healthcare
Coordinate investments, decisions, and policies across CDC and with partners
Make data sharing easier through common policies, practices, and standards
Advance academic and private partnerships
Increased collaboration, communication, and messaging among CDC and partners
Reduced data collection and reporting burden at state, tribal, local, and territorial levels
Improved data sharing and interoperability through common standards like HL7® FHIR®
Increased capacity to quickly analyze, interpret, and act on data
Effective coordination on complex health and emergency response challenges
Timely and complete data reporting to CDC
Efficient, secure data access and exchange between systems across the country
A more comprehensive picture to improve decision-making and protect health for all
ACCELERATE DATA FOR ACTION
Identify data for priority public health needs
Upgrade and modernize IT infrastructure
Strengthen the data science workforce
Adopt open standards and tools while protecting data security
Translate data into evidence-based recommendations
Increased electronic reporting and specific enhancements to flagship CDC surveillance systems
Stronger workforce in data science, analytics, modeling, and informatics
Targeted real-time communication of data and results
Real-time, linked systems that recognize threats early to inform timely response
A highly skilled workforce that applies state-of-the-art data skills and tools
High-quality information and guidance to protect people's health
SUPPORT STRATEGIC INNOVATION
Seek partner-driven data solutions
Develop next-generation tools (e.g., modeling, visualization, predictive analysis, machine learning)
Strengthen predictive analytics and forecasting
Integration and use of data from new or non-traditional sources
Improved pathways to explore, develop, and deploy next-generation technologies
Quick, continued data analysis with adjustment of modeling in real time
Open-source, enterprise-level technologies and coordinated systems
New approaches to address present and future threats
CDC can rapidly identify and effectively mitigate emerging threats
Trusted data promotes evidence-based behaviors, interventions, and solutions to protect health
Every American has equal opportunity to attain the highest level of health possible
All people have the right information at the right time to make decisions
Our country is better prepared for, and protected from, all types of public health threats

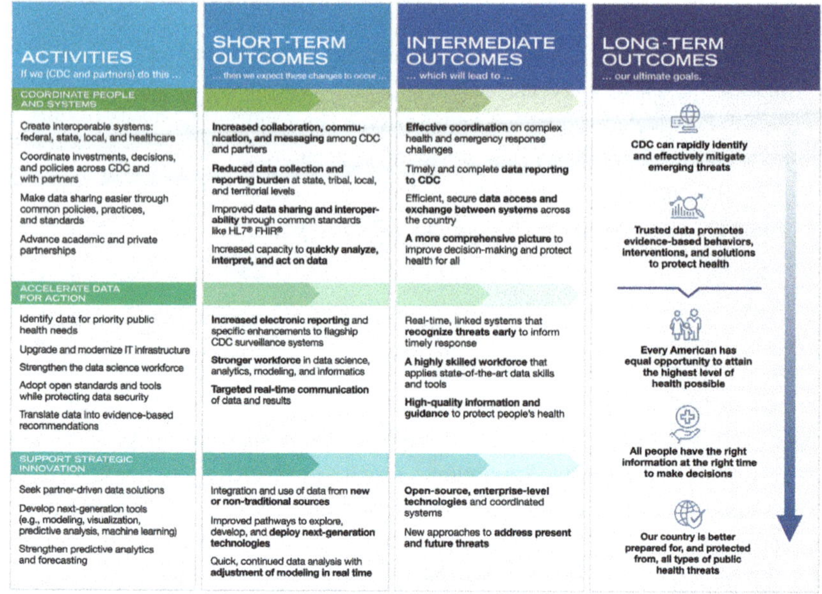

Figure 1. CDC Data Modernization Initiative; a Roadmap of Activities and Expected Outcomes

public health agency to protect the health of all Americans and ensure the stability of the broader world. It is an urgent matter of U.S. national security" (2023). The report focuses on developing and supporting a strong national public health department (Morrison & Inglesby, 2023). It recognizes that during the pandemic, the CDC lost the trust and support of many in the United States. Those in the White House, U.S. Congress, states, and the HHS as well as other stakeholders have agreed that changes are required. It is important that the assessment of CDC consider that the HHS and CDC staff work in collaboration with many across the country. This is an example of a federal department and its agencies that do not stand alone—public health and related policies are collaborative efforts. This important assessment identified the following challenges for the CDC to improve (Morrison & Inglesby, 2023):

- An unclear mission: *A new mission was developed in 2022.*
- An underpowered global mission: *This mission is not understood or valued effectively to ensure Americans are protected from global health threats. Support from policymakers and funding need to be addressed.*
- A diminished independent voice: *This affects the CDC's trusted scientific authority in speaking to the nation.*

- Insufficient presence and leadership in Washington, D.C.: The *CDC is located in Atlanta and thus has limited opportunity for in person contact with HHS staff in Washington.*
- A lack of fully engaged external champions: *The CDC needs partners and coalitions to be more effective.*
- Difficulty recruiting and retaining talent: *The CDC needs to hire better-qualified staff, utilize their expertise, and develop leadership within the agency.*
- An imperative to move at far greater speed: *The pandemic indicated the need to develop a faster response time to crises.*
- A deficit in essential authorities and capabilities: *A critical gap relates to data, coping with a federated system, an antiquated data platform, and issues of privacy, quality, standardization, and predictable and timely access.*

Based on these concerns regarding the CDC's performance, solutions to improve should focus on the following four areas (Morrison & Inglesby, 2023):

1. Develop reorganization plan to elevate core capacities and break down silos; reduce team isolation.
2. Make internal process changes, improving accountability, collaboration, communication, and timeliness across CDC functions.
3. Use a policy framework to improve how the CDC translates its science into guidance and communication, improving the quality and transparency of consultations with external stakeholders.
4. Identify key authorities, budget, and flexibilities essential to acquire data in a timely fashion; hire, deploy, and fund staff; and develop rapid partnerships with private-sector firms.

In summary, the CDC is a key health player in the government that serves as a direct policymaker or provides information and guidance for other policymakers, both public and private. Some of these policies relate to specific diseases and health needs, such as chronic diseases, Alzheimer's disease, and heart disease and stroke; emergency preparedness and response; environmental health; health disparities; immunizations/vaccinations; communicable diseases; health IT; health quality; injury and violence prevention (e.g., occupational safety, suicide, child safety, highway safety, gun violence); reproductive health; smoking and tobacco use; and the healthcare workforce. These areas serve as examples of the many areas that require public policies concerned with health for all levels of government (CDC, 2023a). The CDC is engaged in research, the collection and analysis of data, the sharing of information and resources, the development of legislation and regulations associated with specific policies, the seeking and support of funding, and performance evaluation. These activities affect public policies throughout the CDC, throughout the HHS, and in the healthcare delivery system, both in acute care and public health. As described in **Exhibit 1**, other HHS agencies are also involved in many of these public health activities, and they develop or implement public health policies, running the coordinated services and resources that the HHS provides for national public health.

Public Health: Not a Simple Policy Issue

In 2021, due to the public health crisis, the country experienced political, healthcare, and scientific conflicts as it determined the best responses to the pandemic. This led to public arguments and media expansion on the topic, with many stakeholders engaged in the discussion. At times, it was emotional and threatening. Public health policy and public health were key issues, more so than in the past. The situation demonstrated that public health is important and affects all citizens, government levels, businesses and the economy, healthcare providers and organizations, social services, third-party payers, as well as others; however, it can also lead to conflict. Not everyone views public health in the same manner, and this had an impact on the environment during a time when the importance of public health was stressed. Economic factors also affected the public's response, such as the loss of jobs, reduced work hours, and even increase tuition costs. An example of the latter issue resulted in legal action, which was the case with the University of Delaware. A class-action case was brought due to the cancellation of in-person classes, with concern about differences in cost—typically, in-person classes had different tuition fees from those for online courses. This case was settled with monies going to students who had this experience (Chase, 2023). The cancellation of school and use of online methods was criticized by some in communities and led to disagreements. Throughout the pandemic, policies were challenged legally, increasing the stress, and this has continued post-pandemic.

By 2023, more than half of U.S. states passed legislation related to public health and the pandemic, and some states and communities limited public activities, which was not always accepted, as was noted in the University of Delaware case. One of the laws proposed limited public health authority, affecting the effectiveness of the work that public health officials do and resulting in additional conflict (Nelson, 2021). This led to the development of a collaborative organization, known as Act for Public Health, that focuses on protecting the authority of public health agencies by "providing law and policy research, analysis, expertise, and support for public health agencies as they navigate laws or court decisions affecting their ability to protect their communities" (Krueger, 2023). **Public health authority** is "a public health department's legal ability to further public health by using tools such as community engagement, data collection, scientific research, laws and regulations, enforcement, and the many methods of sharing information and guidance with those who need it most" (Act for Public Health, 2023). Act for Public Health provides the public health system with tools needed to intervene in, maintain, and improve the public's health. Public health agencies have the authority and are responsible for preventing disease, protecting people from environmental hazards, responding to disasters, and helping communities recover. Their work requires active participation of mitigation and hazard experts, and their cooperation and collaboration can improve community resilience to cope effectively.

Since 2006, multiple federal laws (policies) have mandated that the HHS take actions to improve **situational awareness** of threats related to public health emergencies in the United States. The COVID-19 pandemic is an example of the need for this type of approach. These laws require the HHS to develop and implement a near-real-time electronic nationwide public health situational awareness capability using an interoperable network of systems that provide effective technological support. The purpose of this network of systems is to facilitate the early detection of and rapid response to potentially major infectious disease outbreaks, but during the COVID-19 pandemic, it was clear that the 2006 mandate had not yet been adequately met. In 2019, after a review of outcomes from the 2006 law and policy, new legislation, the Pandemic and All-Hazards Preparedness and Advancing Innovation Act (PAHPA), was proposed. This bill repeated the requirement that the HHS improve situational awareness capabilities. This is an example of how policy is not always effectively applied and may need to be changed or be repeated in new policy (HHS, 2023c).

The assessment that guided the 2019 legislation and policy identified the following actions that should be taken by the HHS to develop public health situational awareness and **biosurveillance**, or surveillance/monitoring focused on prevention to detect and respond to biological threats. Both approaches must be part of routine public health and actively used during public health emergencies, focusing on the following (GAO, 2022):

- Designating lead operational division for implementation of statutory requirements and clearly defining its roles and responsibilities
- Identifying the office responsible for overseeing the completion of the activities performed by the lead operational division and clearly defining its roles and responsibilities

- Committing to a deadline for finalizing the work plan to implement the 2019 act requirements and ensuring that the work plan is fully implemented
- Identifying and documenting information to share challenges and lessons learned from the COVID-19 pandemic
- Sharing the lessons learned from the COVID-19 pandemic with relevant stakeholders, such as state, territorial, and local public health officials
- Incorporating lessons learned from the COVID-19 pandemic into plans for implementing the situational awareness and biosurveillance network

How did the HHS respond to this assessment report, the bill, and the recommendations? It agreed to implement 10 of the 12 recommendations and review two of them. The two recommendations that had not yet been accepted and were under review were to identify the office responsible for overseeing the completion of the activities performed by the lead HHS operational division and identify and document information-sharing challenges and lessons learned from COVID-19. It is significant that the content of this report and its recommendations considered feedback from 30 states that responded to questions about what they had learned from the pandemic experience, feedback that provided extensive stakeholder information for policy development. Three common items mentioned in this feedback were as follows (GAO, 2022):

1. Improve public health reporting by, for example, standardizing and sharing data among federal entities and states to improve surveillance needs.
2. Collaborate early with stakeholders by, for example, involving state and local stakeholders throughout the entirety of emergency response activities.
3. Establish a public health infrastructure to enable data sharing by, for example, implementing the network required by the 2019 act.

These suggestions, which emphasize information sharing and collaboration, are integrated into the GAO recommendations listed above and are basic needs for effective public health services. **Figure 2** describes public health situational awareness and the integration of information from various stakeholders and demonstrates the complexity of public health policymaking.

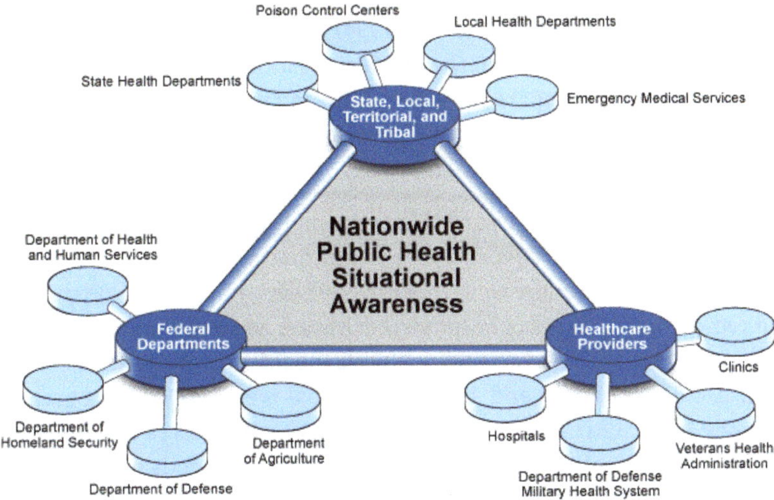

Figure 2. Types of Entities That Must Share Information to Support Nationwide Public Health Situational Awareness

State and Local Governments: Impact on Public Health Policy

State health departments are returning to following routine public health activities after the pandemic. How do they feel about the recent experience public health emergency and its impact (Benadjaoud & Romero, 2023)? Many health departments note that the experience led them to further develop their operational infrastructure, which they view as improved. They, however, are concerned about budget reductions and impact of workforce shortages, which are factors that are likely to negatively impact public health and changes made. States and local governments also must recognize potential future threats, which include infectious diseases and other crises such as the impact of climate change that can lead to weather disasters and public health emergencies. Workforce shortage is a major concern that states have, and if there are other public health emergencies, these shortages can be difficult to handle. In addition, public health departments realize that current staff and future staff need better preparation to provide effective public health services in general and during public health emergencies. In response to these concerns among the states, in March 2023, the American Hospital Association (AHA) made a request to Congress:

> to reauthorize the Pandemic and All-Hazards Preparedness Act (PAHPA: Public Law No. 109417), which was first passed in 2006, to strengthen the Strategic National Stockpile, fund the Hospital Preparedness Program, and require more collaboration between the federal government and stakeholders to build national data infrastructure. (AHA, 2023a)

This law represents a policy, and it is an example of how a healthcare professional organization can advocate for a policy that affects health and services. The AHA is a significant private (nongovernmental) healthcare organization that represents "all types of hospitals, healthcare networks, and their patients and communities. Nearly 5,000 hospitals, health care systems, networks, other providers of care and 43,000 individual members come together to form the AHA" (AHA, 2023b). The organization advocates and lobbies for effective health policy related to a variety of health needs and services in both acute care and public health. The PAHPA is also an example of how a law can be reauthorized to facilitate its application.

To demonstrate collaboration, coordination, and partnership within the HHS in examining and developing policy responses, HRSA representatives, the HHS, state public health representatives, and HHS Secretary Xavier Becerra met with state officials and other partners (HRSA, 2023b). The meeting focused on identifying resources and other supports that HRSA and HHS should provide to state governments and other partners to ensure continuous Medicaid enrollment as policies change or revert to those used prior to the COVID-19 public health emergency. It is critical to continue these partnerships with federal, state, and local government post-pandemic, applying what was learned, continuing to apply effective activities, and considering future needs. Policy needs change, but it is important to ensure that when changes are made, they do not damage public health and ongoing needs at all levels—local, state, and federal.

Global Health and Policies

International health policy has become more important. Situations that are of particular concern for public policy include communicable diseases such as COVID-19, Zika virus, and monkeypox; weather-related disasters, such as floods and fires; earthquakes; and conflict and war, which lead to an increase in the number of refugees and the need for more health services, sheltering, and water sustainability and nutrition. This all requires global surveillance, research, funding, and sharing of information in a manner that is helpful to all countries in need of this information to ensure global public health, with guidance by policies developed by individual countries as well as global organizations such as the WHO and the United Nations. In addition to global emergencies and crises, there also exists the need to address health prevention and treatment, chronic illness, population health management, health services (e.g., medications, provider training and education, universal health coverage, funding), health research, and the impact of the **social determinants of health** (SDOH), which are discussed later in this content. The WHO "leads and champions global efforts to achieve better health for all. By connecting countries, people, and partners, we strive to give everyone, everywhere an equal chance at a safe and healthy life" (WHO, 2023a). Global policy development must look ahead to prepare for health situations that may occur in the future and require cooperation and assistance from multiple countries. The WHO now supports this, with the organization's director's announcement of an initiative to develop and implement a global network to monitor disease threats (WHO, 2023b). The lack of surveillance activity or limited monitoring led to severe problems with the COVID-19 pandemic, specifically in identifying how it started as well as when and where and monitoring its distribution globally over time. With increased travel and connections, globally infectious diseases can be spread quickly without it being recognized. The WHO initiated the International Pathogen Surveillance Network to support its policies about global collaboration. This initiative provides all countries with access to pathogen genomic sequencing and analytics that can be integrated in each country's public health system. This is a global policy decision that will affect current and future policies in many countries to ensure more effective, more timely, more accurate, and higher-quality data on which to base public health decisions and hopefully improve collaboration, coordination, and communication.

Population Health Management and Public Policy: Impact of COVID-19

What is **population health**? It is "the health outcome of a group of individuals, including the distribution of such outcomes within the group" (Kindig & Stoddart, 2003, p. 367). Identified populations, who may be represented by a community (e.g., a neighborhood, town, city, or county) or may represent a segment of a community, are a group of people who share common characteristics (e.g., culture, age, clinical condition, type of residence, and economic factors). Population health must consider diversity and meet various needs. As discussed in this content, the healthcare delivery system, acute care and public health, and the government have recognized the importance of considering Black, Indigenous, people of color (BIPOC) populations;

supporting **health equity**; and decreasing disparities in healthcare services. Doing so requires policies and health reimbursement that integrate health equity, promote inclusion within healthcare professionals' education, and increase workforce diversity (Finkelman, 2023a).

In May 2022, President Joe Biden extended the U.S. public health emergency declaration for another 60 days, and in May 2023, he declared that the public health emergency was over (CMS, 2023a). This type of presidential declaration has a major impact on public health policy, including policies that provided support for many people to obtain free COVID-19 vaccines, tests, and treatment. But what happens when this type of policy ends? It is clear that patients will then have to pay more out of pocket, with the amount depending on the type of insurance they have for health services; it may also affect the level of service they can get covered by their insurance. Who will pay for vaccinations? This will vary depending on insurance coverage (e.g., private insurance, Medicare, and Medicaid). What will be the impact on services? As an example, the use of telehealth expanded, and policies related to these services changed. For example, there were adjustments in Medicare:

> rules governing telehealth so that many more beneficiaries can access such services during the declaration. Telehealth services are no longer limited just to those living in rural areas, and enrollees can conduct visits at home, rather than having to travel to a health care facility, and they receive a wider array of services via telehealth. These flexibilities will end for most beneficiaries after the emergency expires. (Collins & Luhby, 2022)

This demonstrates how the federal government—in this case, CMS—makes policy changes that directly affect the services and reimbursement provided, adjustments that the public will notice. Population health experiences are affected when policies are changed or new guidelines are introduced, and population health management must recognize the relevance of policies as directives, plans, and courses of action required by law (Bhattacharya & Bhatt, 2017). The principles of population health policy must be integrated into public health, which requires consideration of preventive health care; early detection, treatment, and mitigation; and rehabilitation. Political, economic, epidemiological, ethical, behavioral, and legal factors influence the development of policies that relate to population health.

The AHA framework on population heath improvement and management recognizes the need for commitment to access, health, innovation, and affordability. This requires an understanding of populations, leadership, advocacy, change, an expansion of knowledge and sharing (e.g., using evidence-based practice), and measurement and monitoring of needs and outcomes (AHA, 2020; Finkelman, 2023b). The population health management process is applied by healthcare providers, policymakers, and services and includes the following steps:

- Define the focus population.
- Identify core gaps in health and care.
- Stratify risks for the population including consideration of the SDOH.
- Develop a plan identifying interventions and timeline.
- Engage providers and patients in the process.
- Manage care as needed.
- Track and evaluate outcomes using the analysis results to improve.

This process requires the involvement of many stakeholders from local, state, and federal government agencies and their staff and is guided by policies and legislation. Funding for these services is provided by the government, donations and grants, and health insurance reimbursement for services. Along with the various stakeholders, consumers should also be involved to provide feedback and participate in decisions about their needs and health care. As has been noted, needs and policies change, as do communities and populations, requiring adaptation.

As a major source of public health guidance, the HHS recognizes the importance of population health in many of its activities. For example, the CDC:

> views population health as an interdisciplinary, customizable approach that allows health departments to connect practice to policy for change to happen locally. This approach utilizes non-traditional partnerships among different sectors of the community—public health, industry, academia, health care, local government entities, etc.—to achieve positive health outcomes. Population health brings significant health concerns into focus and addresses ways that resources can be allocated to overcome the problems that drive poor health conditions in the population external icon. (CDC, 2020)

The HHS' and CDC's view of population health has an impact on policies related to health and social needs. To support this perspective, the CDC's Division of Population Health (DPH) is engaged in many population health activities, such as prevention strategies for specific populations and settings, support and facilitation of the development and use of innovative public health programs, and data analytics. In addition, the CDC division supports prevention research to better ensure the use of evidence-based practices in population health (CDC, DPH, 2021).

Integration of Equity and Other Related Factors in Public and Community Health Policy

There are many factors that affect the need for policies, their content, and their implementation. The following discussion highlights critical factors that are currently highlighted in policy development to ensure an effective, accessible healthcare system for acute care and public health.

Diversity, Equity, Inclusion, and Accessibility

Diversity, equity, inclusion, and accessibility (DEIA) have become critical elements in effective healthcare delivery and outcomes. Communities are usually diverse, a factor that affects their approach to public health. With increasing concern about disparities in health care, discrimination, and the need to support human rights, healthcare policies now address DEIA through both new policies and a review of current guidelines. Government at all levels is integrating DEIA factors into its structure and functions. The CDC defines ***health equity*** as the "state in which everyone has a fair and just opportunity to attain their highest level of health" (2023a).

The HHS strongly supports advancing health equity, as demonstrated by its equity action plan, which applies to all its agencies (HHS, 2022a). In support of the agency's policy on health equity, the AHRQ published a report about its Consumer Assessment of Healthcare Providers and Systems (CAHPS®) 2022 virtual research meeting, titled *Assessing Patient Experience for Insights Into Enhancing Equity in Healthcare*. The report, which discussed the meeting findings, identified the following key issues (AHRQ, 2022a):

- Disparities exist in the patient experience of racial and ethnic minorities, individuals with limited English proficiency, sexual and gender minorities, and people with disabilities, among others, but there are gaps in our understanding of different population groups.
- Two challenges in measuring the patient experience in these different groups are small sample sizes and low response rates.
- Many individuals have multiple characteristics.
- There is a need for disaggregated data to support a more granular look at subgroups.
- Provider education and training are needed to convey the benefits of collecting demographic data for quality improvement purposes,

Agency for Healthcare Research and Quality (AHRQ), Selection from "Consumer Assessment of Healthcare Providers and Systems (CAHPS®) 2022 Virtual Research Meeting Summary: Assessing Patient Experience for Insights into Enhancing Equity in Healthcare," 2022, p. 2.

mitigating disparities in patient experience among minorities, and communicating sensitively with patients of various backgrounds.
- Measuring structural bias and structural barriers in health care requires complex methodologies to accurately identify, adopt, and implement equity improvement interventions.

Why is this type of government information important within a discussion about public policy? Each of the key issues could relate to policies; for example, a public health department might consider these challenges while assessing its services and plan for improvement. Changes may be needed, and these may require the use of clear policies, such as local or state legislation or application of federal health policies. Provider education and training may be influenced by academic healthcare profession education policies such as education standards (e.g., the American Association of Colleges of Nursing [AACN; 2021]).

The following is an example from the HHS of how policy affects decisions and plans:

> In the context of HHS, this Strategic Plan adopts the definition of *underserved communities* listed in Executive Order 13985: Advancing Racial Equity and Support for Underserved Communities through the Federal Government to refer to populations sharing a particular characteristic, as well as geographic communities, who have been systematically denied a full opportunity to participate in aspects of economic, social, and civic life. This definition includes individuals who belong to underserved communities that have been denied such treatment, such as Black, Latino, and Indigenous and Native American persons, Asian Americans and Pacific Islanders and other persons of color; members of religious minorities; lesbian, gay, bisexual, transgender, and queer (LGBTQ+) persons; persons with disabilities; persons who live in rural areas; and persons otherwise adversely affected by persistent poverty or inequality. Individuals may belong to more than one underserved community and face intersecting barriers. This definition applies to the terms *underserved communities* and *underserved populations* throughout this Strategic Plan. (HHS, 2022b; *Federal Register*, 2021)

This example illustrates how policies are guided by regulation or an executive order.

Private organizations are also engaged in supporting health equity and related factors. The APHA recognizes that:

> these inequities are the result of policies and practices that create an unequal distribution of money, power and resources among communities based on race, class, gender, place, and other factors. To assure that everyone has the opportunity to attain their highest level of health, we must address the social determinants of health AND equity. (APHA, 2021)

Addressing health equity within the healthcare system requires assessment and surveillance, interventions, and evaluation of outcomes (Finkelman, 2023a). Associated is the need for public policy that supports equity. This policy may relate to the types of services provided as well as to and by whom, funding and reimbursement, standards (quality and safety), healthcare professional education, regulations and laws, and research. Equity is now considered a critical factor by government, healthcare professionals and organizations, third-party payers, and other stakeholders and should be considered when new guidelines are developed.

Social Determinants of Health (SDOH)

The report titled *Integrating Social Care Into the Delivery of Health Care: Moving Upstream to Improve the Nation's Health* supports the view that the SDOH represent important aspects of health and healthcare outcomes that require strategies and interventions not directly related to a clinical encounter (NAM, 2019). The report discusses the need for an upstream approach that focuses on SDOH factors that include social-structural influences affecting health; social inequities (e.g., class, race/ethnicity, immigration, gender, sexual orientation); institutional inequities within work and educational settings and government; laws and policies; and living conditions. In the past, the SDOH were not often considered during health planning; however, today there exists greater recognition that this must be done to reach effective outcomes and mitigate social risk factors and/or adverse social determinants (Finkelman, 2023a; 2023b). The **upstream-midstream-downstream public health model** is discussed in greater detail later in the content that discusses policy development.

The SDOH, health equity, and health literacy are included in the Healthy People 2030 initiative (see **Appendix B**). The initiative includes data-driven national objectives related to five SDOH areas: healthcare access and quality, education access and quality, social and community context, economic stability, and neighborhood and the built environment. **Figure 3** describes how the SDOH, equity, and the Healthy People initiative are connected. Some

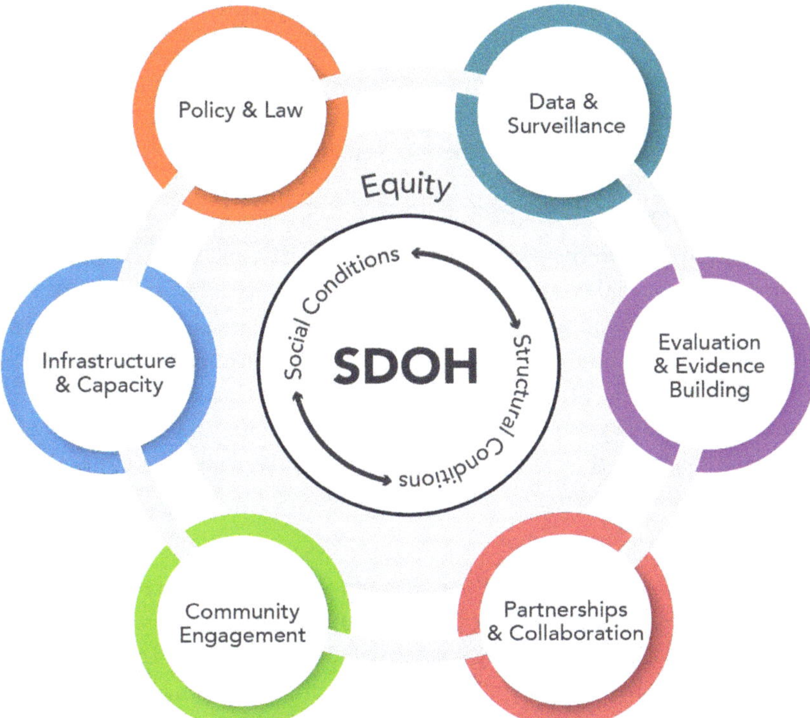

Figure 3. Social Determinants of Health

examples of the SDOH monitored by Healthy People 2030 include safe housing, transportation, and neighborhoods; polluted air and water; and access to nutritious foods and physical health opportunities (CDC, 2022b; 2022c). The data can then be used at the local, state, and federal levels to determine policies and how best to implement them to ensure public health, which is influenced by many factors, including the SDOH, that may not always be associated with health.

As part of the HHS' strategic approach to addressing the SDOH, individuals, regardless of their social circumstances, must have "access to aligned health and social care systems that achieve equitable outcomes through high-quality, affordable, person-centered care" (Chappel, et al., 2022). What can be done to meet this goal, which requires partnerships with active community involvement—including the community, public health system, and community-based organizations? Activities should be associated with collecting and analyzing data, effective financial infrastructure, technology, and the provision of a sufficient and trained workforce, both clinical and nonclinical, to meet health and social needs, recognizing that

that these are interrelated, as illustrated in **Figure 3**. This approach may be referred to as *hubs* or *backbone organizations* and may include participation by governmental and nongovernmental organizations as funders, participants, and other stakeholders. This requires effective collaboration with local public health departments to ensure that the SDOH are included in community population health strategies at all levels of need (Chappel et al., 2022). Policies, plans, and interventions also must consider the impact of stigma in the community. "Stigma, driven by upstream factors connected to social control, is an inherently structural phenomenon with significant health implications. Because laws are powerful mediators for structural stigma, they are critical levers for anti-stigma work" (Conyers-Tucker et al., 2022). Stigma is a social determinant that is important within healthcare delivery. Public health professionals have an important role in reducing stigma—they need to advise policymakers about its importance and to consider it when public health policies are developed, implemented, and evaluated.

> Stigma causes incalculable human suffering. It intensifies harm against the most vulnerable and marginalized communities. Stigma, driven by upstream factors connected to social control, is an inherently structural phenomenon. Because laws are common and powerful mediators for structural stigma, they are critical levers to reduce stigma. (Conyers-Tucker et al., 2022)

Figure 4 illustrates examples of how the SDOH affect various policy issues and their impact in 5 years.

Consumers

Consumers are important stakeholders in policy development. Recognizing the need to better understand consumers and health policy, the AHRQ's CAHPS® held a virtual meeting to assess patient experience and better understand equity in health care. The meeting identified the following themes and key issues (AHRQ, 2022a):

Key Themes:

- Many inequities exist across sociodemographic groups with respect to access to and quality of health and healthcare services.
- Addressing and eliminating health inequities in patient experiences requires an accurate measurement of differences in care experiences and reporting findings.

→ School-Based Programs to Increase Physical Activity
→ School-Based Violence Prevention
→ Safe Routes to School
→ Motorcycle Injury Prevention
→ Tobacco Control Interventions
→ Access to Clean Syringes
→ Pricing Strategies for Alcohol Products
→ Multi-Component Worksite Obesity Prevention
Counseling and Education
Clinical Interventions
Long Lasting Protective Interventions
Changing the Context
Making the healthy choice the easy choice
Social Determinants of Health
HI-5
→ Early Childhood Education
→ Clean Diesel Bus Fleets
→ Public Transportation System
→ Home Improvement Loans and Grants
→ Earned Income Tax Credits
→ Water Fluoridation
SCHOOL
HEALTH IMPACT IN 5 YEARS

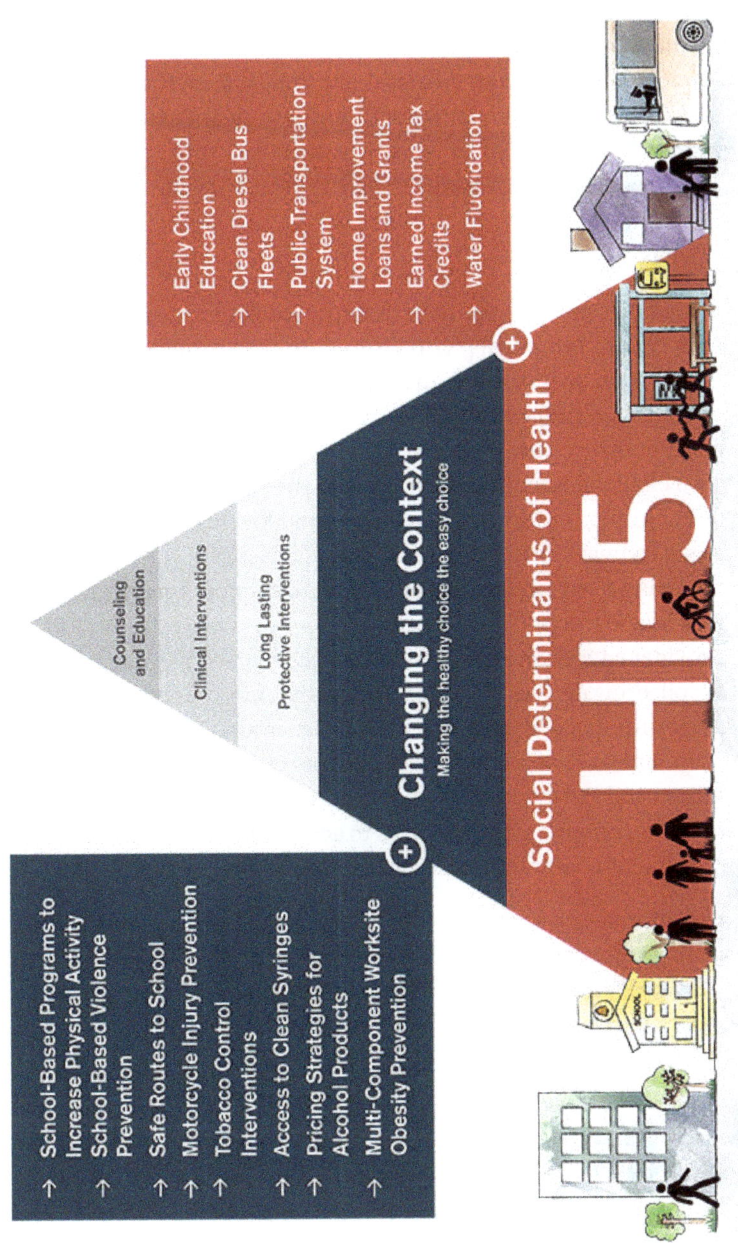

Figure 4. Social Determinants of Health HI-5

- Effectively addressing healthcare inequities requires improvements in data collection and data quality and the use of statistical techniques, such as stratified analyses, to inform quality improvement efforts.
- Producing data that assess health equity and inform equity-targeted quality improvement requires both accurate identification of underserved groups and better response rates from those populations.
- Data should be collected only if there are specific plans to use them.

Key Issues:

- Disparities exist in the patient experience of racial and ethnic minorities, individuals with limited English proficiency, sexual and gender minorities, and people with disabilities, among others, but there are gaps in our understanding of various population groups.
- Two challenges in measuring the patient experience in these different groups are small sample sizes and low response rates.
- Many individuals have multiple characteristics.
- There is a need for disaggregated data to support a more granular look at subgroups.
- Provider education and training are needed to convey the benefits of collecting demographic data for quality improvement purposes, mitigating disparities in patient experience among minorities, and communicating sensitively with patients of different backgrounds.
- Measuring structural bias and structural barriers in health care requires complex methodologies to accurately identify, adopt, and implement equity improvement interventions.

This type of information is useful in providing understanding of important information and evidence to guide policy development—in this case, related to policy and equity based on key stakeholder feedback from consumers, which is important to ensure more effective public health policy.

Health Literacy

Health literacy is an important factor that affects population health, **vulnerable populations**, DEIA, and policy decision (HHS, 2021). The following are definitions of the two health literacy perspectives (CDC, 2021a):

- Personal health literacy is the degree to which individuals can find, understand, and use information and services to inform health-related decisions and actions for themselves and others.

- Organizational health literacy is the degree to which organizations equitably enable individuals to find, understand, and use information and services to inform health-related decisions and actions for themselves and others.

When individuals, populations, and communities understand health information and its implications, they can participate more effectively in personal and public health decisions. Some factors that can act as barriers to health literacy are education, language, culture, technology access and ability, and access to healthcare providers who can share information. Understanding information is an important element, but information also must be applied and used in decision-making.

Of late, there has been greater emphasis on health literacy in policy decisions. For example, the development of the National Culturally and Linguistically Appropriate Services Standards, which are a set of 15 action steps that should be used to advance health equity, improve quality, and help eliminate healthcare disparities by providing a blueprint for individuals and health and healthcare organizations to implement culturally and linguistically appropriate services (Office of Minority Health, 2023). The HHS provides resources and health literacy activities that include the standards and has developed its National Action Plan to Improve Health Literacy. Healthcare organizations and professionals have placed more emphasis on and been influenced by public policy related to health literacy. One example is the ODPHP, a component of the HHS, which developed a research-based guide to help healthcare organizations and professionals design health websites and other digital tools that improve health literacy for individuals, populations, and communities (ODPHP, 2015). These are examples of national policy and actions related to health literacy, but this type of need is also important at the local and state policy levels. Local governments need to ensure that their communities receive and understand clear health information and how it affects public health (e.g., how schools might communicate with parents about overall health prevention for all children in the community or how local health departments share information about immunizations needed by children and adults of all ages).

What can be found in the HHS plan to improve health literacy? Identify several ways in which this plan might influence public health policy.

Website: https://health.gov/our-work/national-health-initiatives/health-literacy/national-action-plan-improve-health-literacy

Nursing Policy: Diversity, Equity, Inclusion, and Accessibility

The report titled *The Future of Nursing 2020–2030. Charting a Path to Achieve Health Equity* (NAM, 2021) examines nursing and its impact on health and healthcare delivery. It notes that community and public health nurses are important in ensuring public health nationally, and nursing should include emphasis on populations that need care and health guidance (e.g., communities of color, communities of lower income, communities with limited access to health care). Preparing nurses to meet these responsibilities requires funding for research and education, which relates to public policy decisions, such as research funding from the National Institute for Nursing Research (NINR). The NINR also supports advancing health equity into the future (NINR, 2023), an aim that is integrated into its structure and functions, annual lecture series, and grants.

The development of the nursing workforce should be monitored to ensure goals are met, and funding from HRSA may assist with workforce improvement. This also requires healthcare organizations to develop their workforce, which requires a consideration of federal, state, and local governments and organizations, and healthcare professional organizations and academic health profession programs standards and policies.

Nursing professional organizations recognize the importance of involvement in all aspects of public policy. The first step is to be aware of current policies and potential changes. These organizations are engaged in private policy and need to share their expertise to ensure that public policy supports the nursing profession and its practice. Nursing organizations have expertise and resources to develop and advocate for DEIA by engaging, educating, and preparing nurses so that they can deliver "patient-centered, culturally responsive care and to effectively recognize and respond to implicit bias in healthcare settings" (Jolley & Peck, 2022). Nursing recognizes that policies need to consider "discrimination due to gender, race/ethnicity, sexual identity, and socio-economic status," which "negatively impacts health of these U.S. populations. Implicit bias (IB) impacts the patient-provider relationship and healthcare outcomes. Efforts are ongoing to define ... IB, identify affected populations, and evaluate provider understanding of IB and its effect on patient care" (Jolley & Peck, 2022).

The following bullets introduce some of the major nursing organizations and their influence and activities related to health policy:

- **AACN:** The AACN participates actively in monitoring policies and engages in offering information to support effective health policies. Its major focus areas are in advancing higher education, pursuing transformative research, developing a robust workforce, and redefining models of care (AACN, 2023). This means that the AACN's focus is on policies that might affect these four areas. The fourth focus, redefine models of care, has a public health emphasis, one that includes supporting models of care for a healthier nation. The AACN also supports investment in community-based centers and public health infrastructure, which leads to accessible, equitable, and affordable population-based care in the community. The organization represents academic nursing programs and has an impact on nursing education policies, standards, and curricula.

- **National League for Nursing (NLN):** The NLN represents nursing education programs and has an impact on nursing education policies, standards, and curricula with its annual development of public policy agendas. These agendas then guide the organization's advocacy related to health policy and in terms of how policy relates to nursing education. The 2023–2024 policy agenda focuses on education (nursing), workforce, access (equitable for individuals, families, populations, and communities), and diversity and inclusion (related to students, the workforce, and patients; NLN, 2023).
- **American Nurses Association (ANA):** The ANA is not directly involved in making legislation (policy) but has an impact through its advocacy for nursing and patients during the policymaking process and implementation of policies at the local, state, and federal levels (ANA, 2023a). The organization works with staff and elected officials in government departments and agencies and routinely monitors the HHS, he CMS, the CDC, AHRQ, the FDA, the HRSA, the Department of Veterans Affairs (VA), and even sections of the government that are not directly associated with health care but that may affect it, such as the Department of Justice, Department of Labor, and Drug Enforcement Agency (ANA, 2023b). The ANA's advocacy empowers nurses and applies influence to improve health for all, and the organization is also concerned with policies related to workforce issues (e.g., licensure and regulation, scope of practice, staff safety, reimbursement, quality improvement, staffing, funding for research, and funding for nursing education). The ANA offers several fellowship programs for nurses to develop understanding and expertise in government relations and health policy, and these programs are associated with public health. One program is the Minority Fellowship, which was initiated to "provide culturally competent care to an increasingly diverse population with ever-expanding needs for mental health and substance abuse disorders services, research, advocacy,

and policy development" (ANA, 2023c). In 2015, the ANA began its Washington Policy Fellowship Program, which is available to all nursing specialties to provide experience in government activities and policymaking (ANA, 2023d). This fellowship is associated with the American Nurses Foundation, the ANA philanthropic entity.

- **American Organization for Nursing Leadership (AONL):** This organization represents nurse leaders and managers and is active in health policy advocacy in all areas of health care and government, supporting active advocacy activities. Examples of key advocacy issues identified by the AONL are promoting workforce programs, elevating nursing research and data, promoting the value of nursing, providing funding for nursing, and supporting the Home Healthcare Planning Improvement Act. This act is important to public health because it supports recognizing advanced practice registered nurses and physician assistants as authorized Medicare providers who may certify patient eligibility for nursing home care. This expands care and provider options (AONL, 2023).

Other healthcare professionals and their organizations are also engaged in similar activities—all advocating for health care (e.g., physicians, pharmacists, social workers, healthcare professional educators).

Development of Policies and the Legislative Process

The CDC is an HHS agency with a major responsibility to collect and analyze data and provide guidance to all levels of government, healthcare professionals and organizations, and consumers to ensure their health. This activity is a critical element in the policymaking process; however, more is needed than just accurate data and information to ensure effective policies. The policymaking process is complex and should be applied effectively. How does this process work? Policies are often associated with laws.

> A law is a tool for protecting and promoting the health of the public. Law has been critical in attaining public health goals, serving as a foundation for governmental public health activities. Many of public health's greatest successes, including high childhood immunization rates, improved motor vehicle safety, safer workplaces, and reduced tooth decay, have relied heavily on law. (CDC, 2023b)

Public health law is relevant today for many areas of health care to ensure equitable services are provided and improve health, such as in areas related to emerging and increasing public health threats (e.g., childhood obesity, health care–associated infections, motor vehicle injuries, violence, mental health, substance use disorder, and prescription drug overdoses).

Policy Development Process

The policy development process is complex, involving many stakeholders and factors that influence the process, content, and outcomes. The issue or problem needs to be identified and understood, which may require collecting data or using data collected for other purposes, data analysis, and identification of key stakeholders. Following a thorough review of the issue, options of interventions or actions are identified. This should include an assessment of costs and benefits—such as whether the options can be effectively implemented, what their impact will be, and the populations whom will be affected.

As the process evolves, politics and advocacy become important. **Politics**, which are a combination of influence and power, must be understood. Consideration should be given to the level of support from elected officials, political parties, businesses, and other stakeholder interests as well as faith-based issues and stakeholders and jurisdictional boundaries (e.g., whether a policy can be applied across state borders, how healthcare professionals and organizations view the policy, and whether they support it). The policy development process is described by the CDC in **Figure 5**.

Policy is a course of action that is followed typically by government as well as by healthcare organizations. The development process may lead to a statute, an ordinance, or a code. Politics and legislation are processes that assist in the development, implementation, and maintenance and review of policies and in establishing programs that need to be provided to citizens, whether at the local, state, or federal level. An example of legislation on a federal level that has had a major impact on health care and the status of health for all U.S. citizens was the 1965 Social Security Act. This law established Medicare, Medicaid, and CMS, which administers these programs. This was a significant law and continues to directly affect large numbers of people who receive this reimbursement and indirectly affect the entire healthcare system. Another significant change was the development of the Healthy People initiative, which was a major policy decision made by the U.S. Surgeon General's office in 1990 and which published its first report in 2000. The initiative reviews health and health care throughout the nation on a 10-year basis with reports provided routinely and major summary reports created every 10 years. The data are used to understand problems

5. Policy Implementation
1. Problem Identification
Stakeholder Engagement and Education
Evaluation
4. Policy Enactment
2. Policy Analysis
3. Strategy and Policy Development

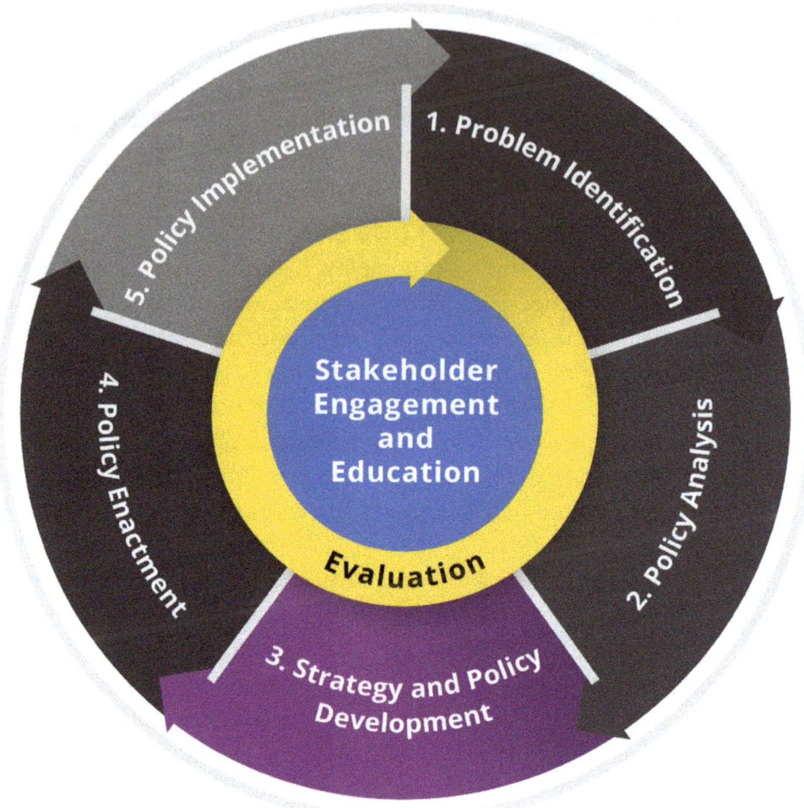

Figure 5. Strategy and Policy Development

and improve care. The current version is Healthy People 2030. More information can be found on this initiative, its reports, and its implications for health policy in **Appendix B**.

The government—all three levels—has a central role in the development and implementation of policies and evaluation of their outcomes. It is important to note that the federal government has limited powers and that state governments have specific powers that may supersede federal powers. State governments are responsible for the public health in their states. There is also an important element in government that needs to be recognized, which is the balance of powers among the three governmental branches. At the federal level, there is the administrative branch, which is associated with the president, other relevant staff, and the presidential administration; the legislative branch, which is the U.S. Congress, elected officials and staff, and its associated offices and departments; and the judicial branch, which begins at the top with the U.S. Supreme Court and includes all levels of the U.S. federal court system. States have similar branches: a governor with associated activities and staff, a legislative branch with elected officials serving in the legislative body and their staff, and a judicial branch with the state system of courts and other judicial activities. Local governments also have similar structures, for example, there may be a mayor, city council, and the local court system that is part of the state system. Local governments and states must collaborate to ensure that state functions and policies are met and collaborate with the federal government.

Legislative Process

The primary method of developing public policy is through the legislative process outlined in Article 1 of the U.S. constitution (U.S. Congress, 2023). It is important when considering policies to understand how a bill, or a proposed law, becomes a law. The **legislative process**, whether at the state or federal level, ensures that specific steps are taken. In addition, even at the local level, decisions are made that are regulations for the community made by the local government. The legislative process is described in **Figure 6.**

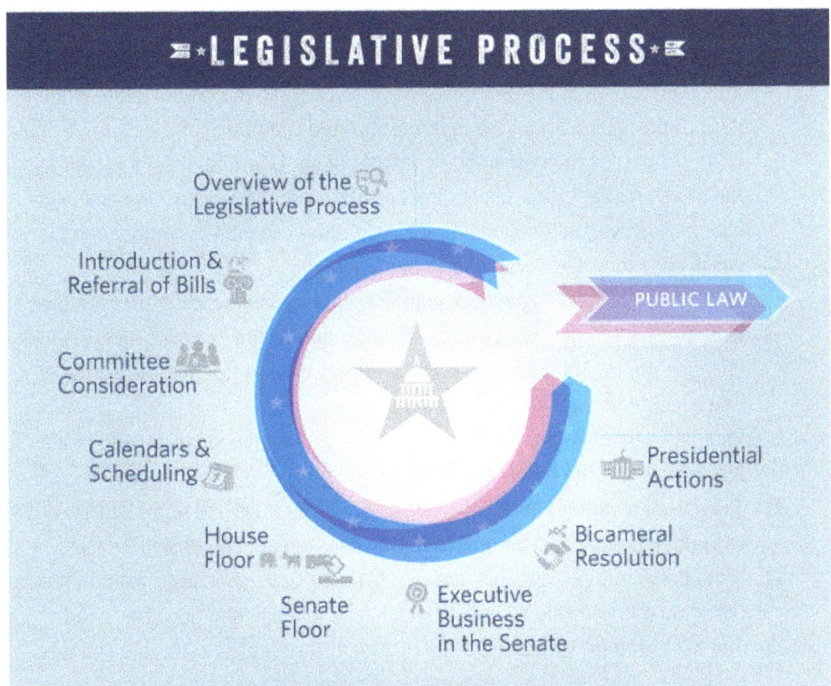

Figure 6. The Legislative Process

Exhibit 3 identifies the steps a bill goes through to become a federal law, associated with the description found in **Figure 6.**

Exhibit 3: From a Bill to a Law

1. A bill, or a proposed law, is developed by either a senator(s) or representative(s); congressional staff assist in the development of the content and assessment of its chance of passage and agreement by the president. During this step, information from experts, research information, comparison with other policies, review of budgetary issues, cost-benefit analysis, assessment of support from healthcare professionals and organizations, identification of political issues and support, and even support at the local and state levels are sought.
2. The bill is then introduced in either chamber of the U.S. Congress by the senator(s) or representative(s) who sponsor(s) it.
3. Once a bill is introduced, the bill, which has a title and number, is assigned to a committee for review, discussion, and even possible changes. The committee should have responsibilities that are associated with the bill's content, such as healthcare policy.
4. If the committee agrees to pass the bill onto a vote in the chamber, it is sent to the associated chamber for a vote (e.g., if a bill was sponsored by a senator, then it goes to the Senate for a vote). A bill can die in committee when it is not passed on for a vote to the associated chamber.
5. If the bill passes the vote in one chamber of the U.S. Congress, it is sent to the other chamber for a similar process of review, discussion, changes, and voting. However, bills can die or not be approved in either chamber vote, in which case they are never sent to the president.
6. Once both chambers vote to accept a bill, there may be differences in the bills that were voted on by each chamber due to the review process and changes made. This requires both chambers to work together to arrive at one acceptable version that both approve.
7. With one version of the bill, both chambers vote on the same version of the bill. If it passes, the bill is sent to the president.
8. The president reviews the bill. The president can approve and sign it into law or can refuse to approve a bill or veto it. This stops the bill, unless Step 9 occurs.
9. If the president vetoes a bill, the U.S. Congress can choose to vote on the bill again and override the presidential veto. The bill then becomes a law.
10. The bill is vetoed by default if the president does not sign the bill and it is unsigned when the U.S. Congress is out of session. This is a pocket veto, and it cannot be overridden by congressional vote.

Policy analysis is a crucial part of the policymaking process. This involves recognizing that some policy decisions may have negative consequences for certain people and communities. Compromises are made that require an examination of costs and benefits to determine the best approach. After evaluation, there may be decisions that need to be changed due to the evaluation data that were collected, presented, and analyzed. Fairness, justice, and equity should be reviewed during the analysis as they are important factors that have an impact on outcomes and should be part of the legislative process.

After a bill is passed and signed, the law is then sent for review by the administrative agency or agencies associated with the law's focus. Typically, **regulations** or rules are developed that will guide how the law (policy) will be implemented. For example, a law that focuses on a health policy might be sent be sent to the HHS and the appropriate agencies within that department for review and identification of regulations to ensure that the policy is implemented, budgeted, and evaluated. Often the government department or agency that is preparing regulations asks for feedback from relevant stakeholders. After regulations are completed, the policy/law is enacted and then evaluated as required either by law or by recommendation in the regulations. Three examples of legislation that required the CDC to develop regulations include the following (2023b):

- Health Insurance Portability and Accountability Act of 1996 (HIPAA) Privacy Rule: This law establishes a rule to protect personal health information and gives patients a variety of rights.
- Human Subjects Research Protections: Institutions engaging in most HHS-supported human subject research must have an approved assurance of compliance with protective HHS regulations.
- Health Information Technology for Economic and Clinical Health (HITECH) Act: This act supports the development of a nationwide health IT infrastructure.

An important aspect of health policy development and implementation is that healthcare providers and organizations must be current regarding policies that affect practice and services, whether they work in acute care or public and community health. For example, they need to be alert at all levels of government to changes that might occur and might affect current policies or the need for changes or new policies and also provide expert input in the development and implementation of effective health policy. It is also important to recognize that some health policy has direct implications for healthcare providers, such as funding for education, reimbursement for healthcare services, and legal regulations about practice, that are important to healthcare providers. The same applies to healthcare organizations and includes funding for research and service grants, reimbursement for healthcare services, application of standards, and evaluation of care and quality improvement.

The Public Health Act of 1944 is an example of important legislation that directed health policy and continues to do so. At that time, the law consolidated all existing public health laws into one law, and it has been amended over the years. Examples of how this law has affected public health include the following: establishment of the NIH and support of its ongoing functioning, funding for prevention and primary care services, establishment of rural health clinics, and family planning services. In addition, there is funding for nursing education and other healthcare provider education. This is an important law that has developed public health and over time influenced health policy throughout the healthcare system.

Policy Content

Public and community health requires polices that support the **Triple Aim** and **STEEEP®** and thus should be reflected in policy content. The Triple Aim focuses on improving care, improving health, and reducing cost, with all directed at population health (Institute for Healthcare Improvement [IHI], 2023a). A fourth element related to the aims is now considered important by some experts: health equity, which is discussed in this content as an important issue in healthcare delivery. It is significant that it is now considered relevant to the Triple Aim. These goals should guide the direction of public policies and health. It is important that the Triple Aim be achieved for all due to its emphasis on equity (Wyatt et al., 2016). Associated with the Triple Aim is STEEEP®, which provides the following framework to ensure effective health services and health (AHRQ, 2022b):

- **Safe:** Avoiding harm to patients from the care that is intended to help them
- **Timely:** Reducing waits and sometimes harmful delays for both those who receive and those who give care
- **Effective:** Providing services based on scientific knowledge to all who could benefit and refraining from providing services to those not likely to benefit (avoiding underuse and misuse, respectively)
- **Efficient:** Avoiding waste, including waste of equipment, supplies, ideas, and energy
- **Equitable:** Providing care that does not vary in quality because of personal characteristics such as gender, ethnicity, geographic location, and socioeconomic status
- **Patient (person)-centered:** Providing care that is respectful of and responsive to individual patient preferences, needs, and values and ensuring that patient values guide all clinical decisions

There are several types of policies. Some become laws through the legislative process, whereas some do not but are still considered policies requiring no legislative action. The following are common types:

- **Regulatory policies:** These are restrictive in that they identify requirements that must be followed, and the requirements may have a negative impact on some and positive impact on others. Some of these policies require self-regulation, such as professional standards. *Examples:* HIPAA; gun control.
- **Distributive policies:** These focus on identifying and allocating resources and benefits. *Examples:* food relief such as the Supplemental Nutrition Assistance Program (SNAP) and Women, Infants, and Children (WIC).
- **Redistributive policies:** These focus on moving funds and resources from one entity or population to another, which sometimes leads to conflicts. *Examples:* Medicare and Medicaid, Temporary Assistance for Needy Families.
- **Incremental policies:** These policies represent several policies that are related to one another and may expand the purpose of a policy as well as how it is implemented and for whom. *Examples:* the civil rights movement, application health equity across all federal government functions and structure.
- **Procedural policies:** These describe how functions (e.g., governmental) are implemented. *Examples:* checklist for federal websites and digital services, National Action Plan to Improve Health Literacy.
- **Social regulatory policies:** These focus on complex social and economic issues and are often difficult to develop and implement. *Examples:* child labor laws, environmental laws.
- **Comprehensive policies:** These policies have a major impact on public attitudes and public health. *Examples:* Medicare and Medicaid, the ACA.

Policy content should focus on identifying policy elements that are likely to be effective and address current needs. The **upstream-midstream-downstream model** is a framework applied to public health policy development. Effective development needs to place less emphasis on individual concerns and more on families, populations, and communities. This model supports public health and applies interventions on multiple levels (Brownson et al., 2010). The following three levels are part of this model (Finkelman, 2023b):

- *Upstream interventions* include the development, implementation, and evaluation of policies focused on populations and related to structural determinants, such as social status, income, racism, and exclusion.

- *Midstream interventions* are implemented within organizations, such as clinics, and are often associated with SDOH (e.g., housing, employment, and food security).
- *Downstream interventions* often focus on immediate health needs and prevention or disease management.

The CMS is active in developing, implementing, and evaluating public health policy so that it can meet its mission. One example of the application of upstream interventions is its activities related to the Accountable Health Communities (AHC) model, which was developed to respond to an identified:

> gap between clinical care and community services in the current health care delivery system by testing whether systematically identifying and addressing the health-related social needs of Medicare and Medicaid beneficiaries' through screening, referral, and community navigation services will impact health care costs and reduce health care utilization. (CMS, 2023b)

The CMS provides resources to support clinical sites that use this model and assesses their outcomes for CMS beneficiaries. The AHC model provides support to beneficiaries with navigation services to meet health-related social needs, such as housing, transportation, food, and safety. Evidence supports the need for this type of model, and the initiative with its related policy was established and funded by the federal government to better understand the gap and interventions to resolve the problems through partnerships that engage health care, public health, social services, other local partners, and residents (Mittmann et al., 2022). The AHC model is connected to meeting the SDOH and ensuring health equity.

Policy Evaluation and Outcome

Evaluation of policy outcomes should be part of the policy development process to determine policy outcomes for individuals, families, populations, and communities followed by changes that might be required as well as possible future policy needs. This evaluation should be documented. For many government policies, reports are required at specific intervals. These serve as a description of the evaluation and outcomes, including the actions and budget. The reports may be published for many stakeholders and required by government committees and agencies. With the Internet, this information is now more readily available and thus can be applied when appropriate within the healthcare system. What impact has the policy had on individuals, families, populations, communities, and stakeholders who have a strong interest in the policy? For example, how might a CMS policy on Medicare and

Medicaid reimbursement affect third-party payers and healthcare providers who receive CMS reimbursement? Quantitative and qualitative data may be included in evaluation. The data are often collected from many sources over time and then analyzed. Following this, the evaluation information might then guide actions that need to be taken to ensure that reimbursement is provided according to policy.

The HHS requested public comments about its draft strategic plan for FYs 2022 through 2026, which the agency often does during policymaking. Healthcare professionals and organizations have a responsibility to participate in this type of policy review and comment on both content and methods. Strategic plans have an impact on future policy decisions. The policy to ensure the development and implementation of a plan also requires the HHS to evaluate its performance. Its FY 2022 annual performance plan and report is an example of the importance of policy-driven continuous quality improvement (CQI) and recognizes the need for an annual evaluation to ensure that the government's healthcare services meet the goal of ensuring the health and safety of the American public. In addition, the HHS develops and implements a strategic plan every four years to ensure that there is regular assessment and updates to its activities. The goals for the HHS FY 2022–2026 strategic plan are as follows (HHS, 2022b):

- **Goal 1:** Protect and strengthen equitable access to high-quality and affordable healthcare.
- **Goal 2:** Safeguard and improve national and global health conditions and outcomes.
- **Goal 3:** Strengthen social well-being, equity, and economic resilience.
- **Goal 4:** Restore trust and accelerate advancement in science and research for all.
- **Goal 5:** Advance strategic management to build trust, transparency, and accountability.

These goals and their objectives reflect current concerns, including equity, the SDOH, and critical health problems and the COVID-19 pandemic experience. They also emphasize the ongoing need for CQI (performance tracking and evaluation) and research. This plan has a direct impact on public health policies, not only at the national level but also at the state and local levels of government.

The RE-AIM is a framework used to evaluate policies and their impacts (Glasgow et al., 2019). The framework's dimensions are reach (R), effectiveness (E), and maintenance (M)—which operate at the individual level (i.e., those who are intended to benefit)—and adoption (A), implementation (I), and maintenance (M), which focus on the staff and setting levels. This framework is one of the most common used to plan and evaluate public health policy and implementation at the local, state, or federal levels or by private organizations (D'Lima et al., 2021).

> Public health is concerned with protecting the health of communities and entire populations (a law, regulation, procedure, administrative action, incentive, or voluntary practice of governments and other institutions). Whether as small as a local neighborhood, or as big as an entire country, policy is one potentially effective way to improve the health of populations. (CDC, 2021a)

As noted earlier in this content, the CDC is very involved in public health policy, and due to this activity, it has developed a policy process that it applies and that is used by other government agencies and departments (federal, state, local), programs and services, research projects, and other organizations. The process includes the following focus areas or domains associated with **Figure 5**. There is a sequence to the process; however, in some situations, the steps may overlap or be implemented in a different order (CDC, 2021b):

1. **Problem identification:** ***Clarify and frame the problem or issue in terms of the effect on population health.*** This requires collecting and analyzing data, defining the characteristics of the problem (e.g., frequency, severity, scope, economic and budgetary impacts) and whom it affects (e.g., age, race/ethnicity, gender, socio-economic status, education level), identifying gaps in data and information, and providing a description that is clear to stakeholders and others.
2. **Policy analysis:** ***Identify different policy options to address the problem/issue; use quantitative and qualitative methods to evaluate the effectiveness, efficiency, and feasibility of the policy options.*** Policy options are described that include a) the health impact of the policy (morbidity and mortality), b) the costs to implement the policy and how the costs compare with the benefits (economic and budgetary impacts), and c) the political and operational factors associated with adoption and implementation (feasibility) and that should be prioritized.
3. **Strategy and policy development:** ***Identify the strategy for getting the policy enacted and how the policy will operate.*** This is a description of how to apply the policy and what is needed for its application, such as engagement of stakeholders and funding. The

Centers of Disease Control and Prevention, Selections from "The CDC Policy Process," https://www.cdc.gov/policy/polaris/training/policy-process/index.html, 2021.

policy (law, regulation, procedures, actions, etc.) is drafted to share with stakeholders for feedback.

4. **Policy enactment:** ***Follow internal or external procedures for getting policy enacted or passed.*** Enact laws, regulations, procedures, administrative actions, incentives, or voluntary practice. Monitor and track the application of this work and application of the policy is important.
5. **Policy implementation:** ***Translate the enacted policy into action, monitor uptake, and ensure full implementation.*** The policy is translated into practice, and standards are defined for implementation of regulations, guidelines, recommendations, directives, and organizational policies; indicators and metrics to evaluate implementation and impact of the policy are identified; resources are coordinated and personnel are trained to implement policy; implementation is assessed, and compliance with and sustainment of the policy for a required period of time are ensured.
6. **Stakeholder engagement and education:** ***Identify and connect with decision-makers, partners, those affected by the policy, and the general public.*** Engagement and feedback are obtained.
7. **Evaluation:** ***Formally evaluate the appropriate steps of the policy cycle, including the impact and outcomes of the policy.*** Evaluation needs, purpose, and intended users are defined; evaluation is implemented; and results are shared.

This process should be familiar to healthcare providers as it is similar the healthcare process (e.g., the nursing process). The process can also be applied to the legislative process described earlier in **Figure 6**.

Policymaking should include the development of a written **policy brief**, which is a clear statement of evidence about a policy issue used to clarify a policy and other aspects of its implementation. There are four common types of policy briefs (CDC, 2021c):

1. ***Information brief:*** Provides a summary of the research on a policy method, approach, or other related topic such as behavioral economics or the HiAP approach.
2. ***Issue brief:*** Provides a summary of the best available evidence on a public health problem with policy implications. This type of brief is best used when there are no known policy solutions and the issue is still in the problem identification domain of the policy process.
3. ***Policy brief:*** This type of brief provides a summary of evidence-based best practices or policy options for a public health problem. It is appropriate for issues in domains 2, 3, 4, and 5 of the policy process:

policy analysis, strategy and policy development, policy enactment, and policy implementation, respectively.

4. ***Policy impact brief*:** This is the most in-depth briefing document and includes a summary of the best available evidence on the health, economic, or budgetary impact of one or more policies for a public health problem; it is used when evaluations and evidence exist related to the health or economic impact of the policy.

See **Figure 7** describing the four types of briefs.

The steps used by policymakers to develop a written policy brief are as follows (CDC, 2021c):

1. Identify your audience (who will read or review the brief, receive the content information).
2. Conduct audience research; know your audience.
3. Determine your purpose and make sure your material contains one obvious message.
4. Develop content for the type of brief and define terms, avoid jargon, organize the content in "chunks," and use bullets and other types of formatting to support content flow.
5. Include at least one visual aid that conveys or supports the main message.
6. Format the brief so that it is concise and easy to read.
7. Include considerations for specific audience.

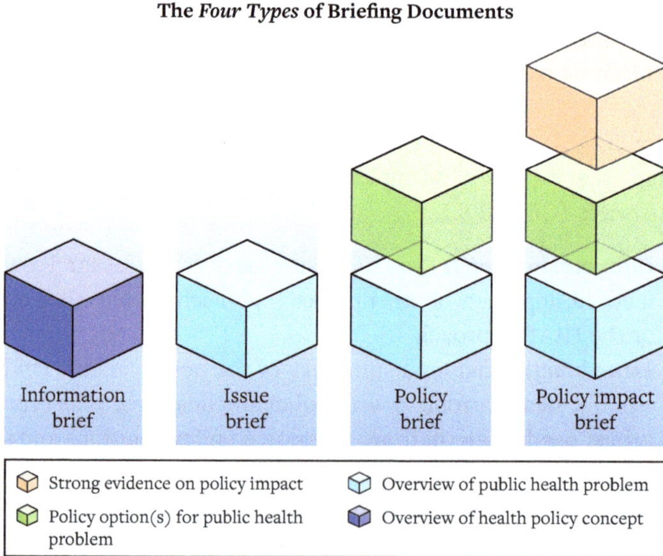

Figure 7. Four Types of Briefing Documents

Political Factors and Healthcare Profession Engagement in Policy Development

Healthcare providers may engage in the policymaking process in a variety of ways and offer their expertise by participating in the political aspects of policy development. Nurses and other healthcare professionals who may work in public and community health may be active participants in identifying the need and content for policies. They may be active change agents within their organizations or their positions, understanding public policy and then applying it.

Advocacy is one activity that providers might use by sharing their expertise to speak for others or support others. As is true for most political activities, they may be done by individuals or groups.

> Beginning health policy advocacy work is a learning process, and we must be prepared to learn as we take our first steps. Those first steps of health policy advocacy may begin along different avenues: consumer groups, workplace settings, nursing organizations, mentor networks, or with elected officials. The steps should be organic and authentic to the individual: phone call, email, letter to the editor of a local newspaper, personalized note to an elected official. (Anders, 2021, p. 92)

Advocacy is a factor related to politics and the legislative process.

Another activity is **lobbying**, or providing expert witness testimony and advocating for consumers to influence a decision or policy. Nurses and other healthcare providers may lobby on an individual or organizational basis. For example the ANA, the American Medical Association (AMA), and the APHA all lobby the U.S. Congress and federal-level departments and agencies. They also lobby at the state level. To influence health policy, one cannot focus solely on the federal level. The state level must also be considered as states have major responsibilities for health, and there can be variations between states and their policies. Professional associations also lobby, and nurses and other healthcare professionals are very active in their own professional organizations. Typically, these organizations have **political action committees** (PACs), which are important organizations using collective action to influence legislation and policy decisions. Examples of organizations that have PACs are the ANA (ANA, 2018) and the AMA. **Coalitions** are another method used by healthcare professionals to influence health policy. This occurs when two or more groups get together or collaborate to use their expertise and resources to meet identified goals. For example, the ANA, the AMA, specialty organizations within nursing or medicine, and the AACN may form coalitions with specific goals in mind that agree with their individual concerns and policy perspectives but also are in sync with others in the coalition.

Professional activities used to influence policies must consider local, state, and federal issues and policies. Throughout this content, there has been discussion about the impact of COVID-19 on policy, and some policies led to new laws at the state and federal levels. An example illustrating federal policy and state policies is the decision by the federal government to support use of the crisis standards during the pandemic and the need for each state to decide whether it would apply those standards. This was a major decision that affected health care for all people within the states (Hick et al., 2021). Healthcare professionals spoke out about the use of the standards, with some supporting them and some opposing. Not all states agreed to use the crisis standards even though they had been recommended. Why was there a conflict over their use? Crisis standards of care may impact who receives care and they type of care that is offered thus some patients may receive limited care (IOM, 2012), These are difficult decisions to make during a time of crisis and increased workload. It may also affect routine healthcare needs and have a long-term negative outcome. Laws are also associated with decisions to declare a public health emergency and the use of some interventions, such as those noted here with the crisis standards.

Healthcare professionals also serve in public offices, whether they are in elected or nonelected positions within local, state, or federal government. This is important as they provide expertise or greater understanding of health and health care to those within the government who may lack this type of information or expertise.

> Nurses are sorely underrepresented in elected office—from local school boards to the halls of the U.S. Congress. Currently [as of 2022], only three nurses serve in the House of Representatives and a nurse has never served in the Senate. The National Conference of State Legislatures tracks state legislators' occupations. Because so few nurses serve in state legislatures, they don't even merit an occupational category; they're included among 'other.' (Summers & Gordon, 2022)

Healthcare professionals also vote in their communities and can affect policy. They may also assist candidates by campaigning for candidates who support certain kinds of health policy decisions or decisions that might affect health. Not all policies important to health care are directly focused on health, such as the SDOH. As discussed earlier, the SDOH need to be included in policy discussions about health as they have implications for legislation regarding housing, nutrition, employment, health reimbursement, and schools even though these issues may not appear to be directly related to health or healthcare services. However, they affect consumer health, how the consumer receives care, public and community health planning, and implementation of public health. Other methods healthcare providers may use to influence policy is to visit their legislative representatives and discuss issues, share expertise in written or oral form, and serve as a resource when needed, providing public presentations about policies. Electronic methods have made it easier for healthcare providers to communicate and try to influence policymaking. Participating in policy fellowships is another method that expands policymaking expertise for healthcare professions. Several examples of these fellowships are discussed in the text.

Implementation of Policies

In response to the need for a more effective public health data system, the CDC established a new center to advance the use of forecasting and outbreak analytics in public health decision-making, known as the Center for Forecasting and Outbreak Analytics (CDC, 2021b). The center includes next-generation public health data, experts in understanding disease causes and trajectories, public health emergency responders, and high-quality communications to meet the needs of decision-makers nationally and at the state level. This will provide more efficient and timely access to information to mitigate the effects of disease threats, such as the social and economic disruption that were experienced during COVID-19. As is true for most new government initiatives, these activities will integrate equity and accessibility and consider innovation and research. The focus of the center's activities is prediction, connection, and information. This is another example of how a public health crisis led to policies and then additional guidelines as more was learned about the crisis and responses.

HiAP is a collaborative model that integrates and identifies the need for health considerations during the policymaking across sectors to improve the health of all communities and people. This model has an impact on effective policy implementation (CDC, 2016). The approach is important as it supports the view of many factors that not considered related to healthcare but that are important to health and public health interventions and programs. HiAP is associated with meeting the National Prevention Strategy and Healthy People goals; representing policies that support state, territorial, and local health departments in improving health outcomes; and assisting in identifying gaps in evidence that is needed for effective public health and to better ensure health equity (see **Figure 8**).

Healthcare professionals have a responsibility not only to engage in policy development but also to ensure policies are implemented in the manner

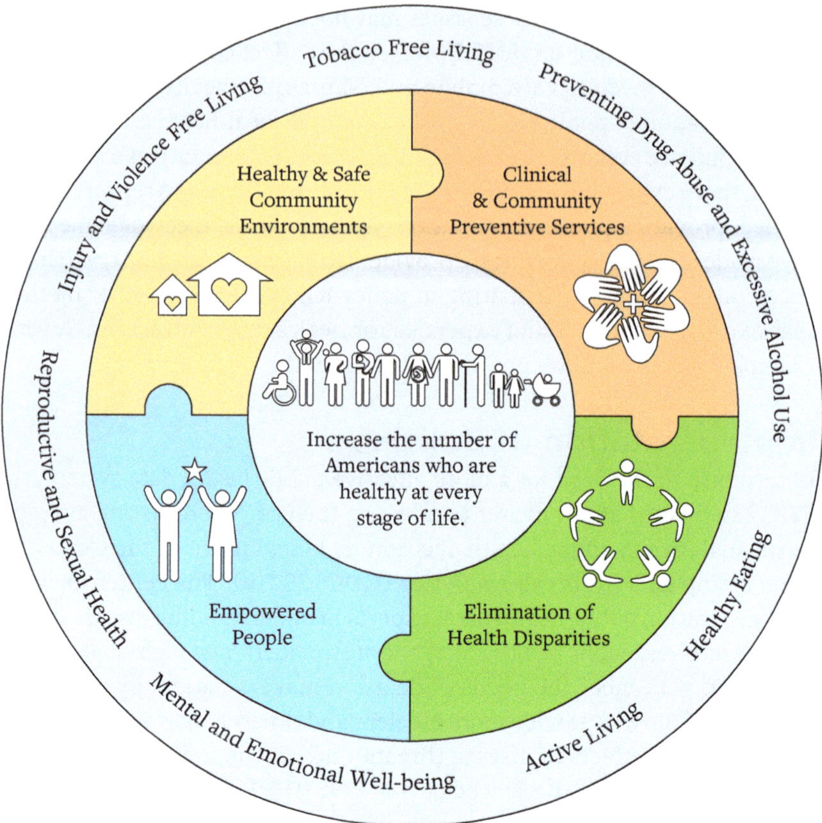

Figure 8. Health in All Policies

expected for them. This requires competencies and understanding. The Council on Linkages Between Academics and Public Health Practice identifies core competencies for public health professionals, which include public health. The following identifies competencies related to Domain 2: Policy development and program planning skills (Council on Linkages Between Academia and Public Health Practice, 2021):

1. Develops policies, programs, and services
2. Implements policies, programs, and services
3. Evaluates policies, programs, services, and organizational performance
4. Improves policies, programs, services, and organizational performance
5. Influences policies, programs, and services external to the organization
6. Engages in organizational strategic planning

Funding and Reimbursement Issues Related to Public and Community Health Policy

Funding and reimbursement are part of policy development, content, implementation, and assessment, regardless of the source or level of government. The following discusses some of the factors that are important in ensuring funds for policies as well as some examples.

Funding and Reimbursement

Developing policies involves expenses for staff, technology, and others; however, when policies are developed, funding is necessary for the implementation and assessment of policy outcomes. If the policy is connected directly to providing healthcare services, reimbursement for them becomes important. Budgets are typically part of policies and legislation. For example, a budget may address costs for establishing a service or program or describe reimbursement for healthcare services.

Health reimbursement is critical to effective public health. Lack of coverage affects access to health services when they are needed. If people have poor coverage and inadequate funds to cover expenses, they may cut back on prescriptions to stretch medication over time, which affects the drug's effectiveness and their health. They may not follow best preventive health measures. There are also issues with missing work due to illness when care is available due to high cost or when there is a need to care for a family member who may not have healthcare coverage. This also affects mental health, family stress, finances for other needs, and other issues, and the SDOH have an impact on outcomes. This can also lead to long-term health problems. Employment is related to these problems since the U.S. health reimbursement system is primarily dependent on employment, and without employment, health reimbursement problems increase.

Federal policies related to healthcare reimbursement are critical and affect national health care and care within states. When these policies change, the transformation can lead to additional problems or improve care by offering more effective reimbursement for health services. An example of a problem associated with a CMS Medicare and Medicaid policy is exceeding the income threshold for Medicaid, which results in loss of coverage.

> The loss of eligibility for Medicaid supplemental insurance above the federal poverty level, which increases cost sharing

> in Medicare, was associated with increased racial and ethnic health care disparities among low-income Medicare beneficiaries. Expanding eligibility for Medicaid supplemental insurance may narrow these disparities. (Roberts et al., 2023, p. 534)

Major legislation that has had an impact on reimbursement is the ACA. It is also an example of the impact the judicial system can have on policies, even those that were created in the past. There was a legal effort to eliminate preventive services from the reimbursement program established by ACA based on a question of constitutionality. The case and decision eliminated the need for health plans to cover preventive services at no cost to patients. This was a significant decision and a problem for consumers and public health. The court decision was appealed, and in June 2023, it was temporarily stayed, meaning that health plans had to return to the original payment requirements for preventive services (Kiff, 2023). It is important to note that this is not a final decision, and it may change again. In addition, the court decision did support exemptions for some health plans to continue with requiring some patient payment due to the health plan's size and other factors, but most must meet ACA's original requirements to cover preventive services. This law may also come up again in other legal cases, and thus legal concerns can be an ongoing threat to policy status.

An example of complex funding and use of resources in policymaking at the federal and state levels occurred during the COVID-19 pandemic. This public health emergency required many new policies and changes to current guidelines (Cubanski et al., 2023). Some were related to healthcare coverage, costs, and payment for COVID-19 testing, treatments, and vaccines; Medicaid coverage and federal match funding; expansion of telehealth and related regulations and reimbursement issues; expansion of Medicaid and the Children's Health Insurance Plan (CHIP) to meet public health needs; private insurance and adjustments; access to medical countermeasures (vaccines, tests, and treatments) and medical equipment through FDA emergency use authorization; liability immunity to administers medical countermeasures; and application of Medicaid Disaster Relief State Plan Amendments. This is complex and requires monitoring and partnerships with states to effectively apply new or changed policies. With so many issues and time a concern, it was also important to manage new policies to ensure that that there was coordination and collaboration—policies needed to be in sync with one another and not limit others.

Funding: Public and Private Grants

Grants are a funding method used to provide funds for specific purposes, most commonly for research but also to support healthcare programs. This funding is provided by government and private organizations as well as individuals. Policies may focus on grants or grants may be part of an overall policy; for example, the establishment of a program in the HHS to provide resources for healthcare services in communities may also include grants to examine interventions (i.e., research). The NIH is the critical part of HHS that focuses on research and grants, providing funding for grants and assessing grant funding outcomes. It is also active in overall policymaking, as demonstrated by the following activities (NIH, 2023a):

- **The NIH Office of Science Policy (OSP)** promotes progress in the biomedical research enterprise through the development of sound and comprehensive policies. The OSP also is the primary policy adviser to the NIH director on matters of significance to the agency, the research community, and the public. The OSP works on a wide range of issues, including biosafety, biosecurity, genetic testing, genomic data sharing, human subject protections, the organization and management of the NIH, and the outputs and value of NIH-funded research. This is accomplished through a wide range of analyses and reports, commentary on emerging policy proposals, and the development of policy proposals for consideration by NIH, the federal government, and the public.
- **The Office of Legislative Policy and Analysis (OLPA)** serves as the principal office within the NIH's Office of the Director and provides legislative analysis, develops policies, and liaises with Congress. The OLPA facilitates and enhances the relationship between NIH and the Congress; advances NIH legislative priorities; and ensures that the NIH community receives essential information, advice, and guidance regarding developments in the Congress that affect the institution.

An example of funding associated with health policy is the NIH-funded study that examined national and state-level estimates of the economic burden of health disparities by race and ethnicity and educational levels, a critical health issue that has had an impact on public health policies (NIH, 2023b). Given that health equity is a major element in public health policy today, this is an important study. The results indicate that the economic burden of health disparities in the United States continues to be very high: In 2018, racial and ethnic health disparities cost the U.S. economy $451 billion, a 41% increase from the 2014 estimate of $320 billion. This study is the first to estimate the total economic burden of health disparities for five racial and ethnic minority groups nationally and for all 50 states and the District of Columbia. It applied a health equity approach and was associated with the Healthy People 2030 goals; used a single standard that can be applied nationally and within each state for all racial, ethnic, and education groups; and estimated the economic burden of health disparities by educational levels as an identifier of socioeconomic status. The researchers concluded that "federal, state, and local policy makers should continue to invest resources to develop research, policies, and practices to eliminate health inequities in the US" (LaVeist et al., 2023, p. 1682). This type of funding provides important data that are needed to examine health issues and develop effective approaches to resolve public health problems; however, it requires funding to complete these activities (e.g., for expertise, data collection and analysis).

Healthcare Spending

Healthcare spending is described in government budgets and assessed routinely by the federal, state, and local governments to determine policy outcomes and manage their funding. The following descriptions are examples of this type of spending that demonstrate the amount of funding can be large:

- Burnout and resilience funding is an example of healthcare spending associated with public health policies. In July 2021, the HHS announced funding of $103 million for the American Rescue Plan to strengthen resiliency and address the problem of healthcare workforce burnout and develop solutions. Workforce issues have been a long-term problem that increased with the pandemic, which led to additional demands on staff and the healthcare system. In addition, staff experienced personal stress and concerns for themselves and their families due to the virus. This type of problem requires nurses and staff to step up, speak out (advocate), and demonstrate leadership to ensure effective implementation of this funding and support this policy. It was thought that these workforce problems would be reduced when the pandemic lessened; however, they were not. This has implications for continuing and funding the policy.
- The Coronavirus Aid, Relief, and Economic Security Act of 2020, also known as the *CARES Act*, is a $2.2 trillion economic stimulus bill (U.S. Department of the Treasury, 2020). This legislation represented a complex policy response to the economic problems

associated with COVID-19 pandemic in the United States. It included stimulus checks to assist citizens during a time of great need and stress related to financial problems due to the loss of jobs, reduced work hours, the loss of benefits, and the financial business losses that affected many people and their families. A lack of funds has a direct impact on health in communities (e.g., on family support, nutrition, safe housing, mental health, crime and violence, substance use disorders). Financial support was also offered to healthcare providers and organizations to ensure that services could be offered. Funding was provided to develop and expand telehealth services so that care could be provided even when patients might not be able to come to a clinic or hospital. Medical testing needed to continue, and the CARES Act helped support this healthcare service.

As an example of complex legislation that established policies and affected funding, examine the health provisions found in the CARES Act.

Website: https://www.kff.org/coronavirus-covid-19/issue-brief/the-coronavirus-aid-relief-and-economic-security-act-summary-of-key-health-provisions/

There is other public health funding that is not directly related to COVID-19 but that focuses on critical issues that need to be addressed—workforce concerns, in particular. The examples, similar to the previous, require high levels of funding. In June 2023, through its agency the HRSA, the HHS announced funding of nearly $9 million to support the preparation of more healthcare providers to assist with the substance use epidemic and the increasing need for mental health services. This funding established the Integrated Substance Use Disorder Training Program, the goal of which was to:

> establish a foundation of skills and expertise for community-based programs and increase the number of nurse practitioners, physician assistants, health service psychologists, counselors, nurses, and social workers who are trained to provide mental health and substance use disorder treatment, including opioid use disorder services. (HHS, 2023d)

At the same time the funding was announced, the HHS announced that $15 million would be provided to recruit and retain clinicians who provide health care to children and adolescents. This initiative focuses on the following:

> In exchange for three years of service working in a health professional shortage area, medically underserved area, or providing care to a medically underserved population, the Pediatric Specialty Loan Repayment Program provides up to $100,000 to eligible clinicians providing pediatric medical subspecialty, pediatric surgical specialty, or child and adolescent behavioral health care, including substance use prevention and treatment services. (HHS, 2023e)

Both examples of funding are associated with policies to support and expand the healthcare workforce and their preparation and services for populations who experience limited access and have complex needs. However, policy like this also requires funding inclusion.

Some policy-related funding is associated with research grants that focus on workforce issues. An example is the HRSA call for grant proposals related to the Nurse Education, Practice, Quality and Retention (NEPQR) Simulation Education Training (SET) program.

> The purpose of the NEPQR-SET program is to enhance nurse education and strengthen the nursing workforce by increasing training opportunities for nursing students through the use of simulation-based technology, including equipment, to increase their readiness to practice upon graduation. This training expands the capacity of nurses to advance the health of patients, families, and communities in rural or medically underserved areas experiencing diseases and conditions such as stroke, heart disease, behavioral health, maternal mortality, HIV/AIDS, and obesity. The goal of the NEPQR-SET program is to increase the number and capacity of nursing students to address the health care needs and improve patient outcomes of rural and/or medically underserved populations. (HRSA, 2023c)

This represents important policy related to healthcare education—in this case, for nurses—and has an impact on practice and meeting workforce preparation needs. This also is a policy and funding issue that would have direct implications on and thus the interest of nursing education organizations.

Uninsured and Underinsured

Providing effective health insurance coverage has long been a public health policy issue. It is a particular concern for people who do not have health insurance (i.e., those who are uninsured) or do not have sufficient coverage to meet their needs (i.e., those who are underinsured). An example of the complexity and impact of this issue occurred in 2020 when some of the Medicaid and CHIP requirements were temporarily waived to reduce the number of people who were losing their healthcare coverage during the COVID-19 pandemic. The policy ended on March 31, 2023. "The expiration of the continuous coverage requirement presents the single largest health coverage transition event since the first open enrollment period of the ACA. Each state has their own process and timeline for asking people who are currently enrolled in Medicaid to demonstrate that they still qualify for Medicaid benefits" (HRSA, 2023d). Some people affected by the change in policy can apply for health plans through the Health Insurance Marketplace associated with the ACA and receive some assistance to cover costs. The following data demonstrate the impact of this type of policy change (i.e., returning to an earlier policy after a temporary adjustment) and loss or limitations in coverage (HRSA, 2023d): A total of 14 million people are patients in health centers covered by Medicaid; 50% of all births in rural, nonmetropolitan areas; and nearly every newborn received newborn screening; however, this is now reduced. In response to these reductions, since the policy is no longer in effect post-pandemic, the HRSA directed $4.5 million to assist with coverage gaps. Health insurance coverage data for 2022 indicate that the following are critical needs (Cohen & Cha, 2022):

- Number of persons younger than age 65 who were uninsured at the time of interview: 27.3 million
- Percentage of persons younger than age 65 who were uninsured at the time of interview: 10.1%
- Percentage of children younger than age 18 who were uninsured at the time of interview: 4.2%
- Percentage of adults ages 18 to 64 who were uninsured at the time of interview: 12.2%

A Major Reimbursement Policy: The Affordable Care Act (ACA)

The ACA represents the most significant healthcare policy in 15 years. It is focused on federal healthcare reimbursement policy that is integrated with states and has had an impact on the number of uninsured people. It provides other options for insurance, reducing the number of those uninsured. CMS has long provided coverage for vulnerable populations, but more assistance was needed, both for the uninsured and to reduce the problem of underinsurance (e.g., some people need to pay more copayments for services or have greater out-of-pocket expenses). The ACA is also an example of a public policy that has not been universally accepted, both when it was proposed and approved and today, as noted earlier when discussing the case that addressed preventive services provisions in this law. Other efforts have been made through the judicial process to alter this law. This is a federal policy, but it has direct implications for states and requires state engagement with the reimbursement program associated with Medicaid, which is connected to states and state policies. The HRSA is responsible for overall management of ACA and implementation of this reimbursement policy.

> Since 2014, when HealthCare.gov was launched, enrollment has doubled from 8 million to more than 16 million. Nearly 16.4 million consumers selected or were automatically re-enrolled in health insurance coverage through HealthCare.gov Marketplaces and State-based Marketplaces (SBMs) during the 2023 open enrollment. Enrollment has increased year-over-year, with 1.8 million more consumers signing up for coverage during the 2023 open enrollment compared to the 2022 open enrollment, a 13% increase, and nearly 4.4 million more consumers signing up compared to the 2021 open enrollment, a 36% increase. (HHS, 2023f)

Research and Evidence-Based Practice Supporting Public Health Policy

Public health research and evaluation of policies need to address the following: "In public health policy, the key question is not just what works, but what works for whom, in what circumstances, and in what ways?" (Sisnowski & Street, 2017). Research is needed to understand public health policy and any gaps that may be present. Results from this research can lead to **evidence-informed health policy** and support **evidence-based practice** (EBP). Just as there is greater emphasis placed on evidence-based care and evidence-based management, policy development needs to focus on evidence-informed public health policy. The government—particularly NIH as well as the NINR—focuses on providing this type of research.

The development of effective new policy and implementation of changes to policies require evidence to support the content and methods. This may be and often is research-based; however, as is the case with EBP, there are other types of evidence that are relevant to policies. Examples are government reports such as the NHQDR and the Healthy People 2030 initiative; expert consultation; data collected for a variety of purposes (e.g., by the CDC, the AHRQ, and others); assessment of outcomes (e.g., programs and services) and standards (e.g., clinical, educational); observations made by experts and healthcare professionals and organizations; and feedback from stakeholders. Two broad categories of evidence are quantitative (numerical) and qualitative (nonnumerical). In some situations, both categories are used.

The AHRQ's mission is to produce evidence to make health care safer, higher-quality, more accessible, more equitable, and more affordable and to work within the HHS and with other partners to ensure that the evidence is understood and used (AHRQ, 2023a). The Center for Evidence and Practice Improvement, which is part of the AHRQ, develops new knowledge, synthesizes evidence, translates science based on what works in health and healthcare delivery, and catalyzes practice improvement across healthcare settings. The following AHRQ divisions assist in developing and evaluating public health policies and provide evidence to support effective policies (AHRQ, 2023b):

1. **EBP Center program:** Produces evidence syntheses by conducting systematic evidence reviews and using robust and rigorous methodologies and advances the methods of evidence synthesis to ensure scientific rigor and unbiased reviews
2. **U.S. Preventive Services Task Force (USPSTF) program:** Provides scientific, administrative, and dissemination support for the independent **USPSTF**, enabling the task force to make evidence-based recommendations about clinical preventive services
3. **Division of Decision Science and Patient Engagement:** Supports informed decision-making by translating evidence-based findings into tools and products that communicate what works in health care; collaborates with stakeholders to promote evidence-based decision-making; and advances research into methods and products that summarize evidence and engage patients, healthcare professionals, policymakers, and communities in improving health care and clinical decision-making
4. **Division of Digital Healthcare Research:** Develops and disseminates evidence to inform policy and practice on how HIT can improve the quality of health care
5. **Division of Practice Improvement:** Advances the science of clinical practice improvement; evaluates and supports innovative models of practice transformation in diverse settings; facilitates communities of learning to promote the implementation of evidence for practice improvement; and serves as a trusted source of evidence and tools for methods, measures, and evaluation of practice improvement.

Policymakers use the resources provided by these divisions to examine the need for policies; create methods to address issues and problems; develop specific policy content; determine how best to implement the policy as well as the best type of policy (e.g., legislation or regulation); and evaluate outcomes. These divisions offer not only informational resources but also expertise to healthcare providers, healthcare organizations, and public and private policymakers.

Review the NINR's featured research topics. Select two and explain how they might relate to public policy.

Website: https://www.ninr.nih.gov/newsandinformation/featured-research

Examples of Current Issues and Their Relationship to Public and Community Health Policy

This content examines several examples of current issues and their relationship to public and community health policy. Included in the examples are public health emergencies; public health nursing and policy; Healthy People 2030 and other major government initiatives that have an impact on health policy; several examples of health problems with major public health implications, including regarding drugs and approvals for public health policy; refugee, immigrant, and migrant workers and public health needs; technology and digital health; and rural health and public policy.

Public Health Emergency

> Policy makers have recognized the need for rigor in public health's emergency (PHEPR) planning and response activities, but while investments have been made in research, this funding has been sporadic, not well coordinated, and not always focused on the needs of public health practitioners. The result has been a relatively sparse evidence base for PHEPR practices, reflecting broad variation in research design, implementation, reporting, synthesis, and translation. (NAM, 2020, p. ix)

Significant investment is needed in the public health system, which includes PHEPR, as demonstrated in this report from the NAM, a nongovernmental, nonprofit organization that provides resources for policymakers. See **Appendix C** for further information about the NAM and its resources.

PHEPR requires a strong social safety net; border policies need to consider risk for infections and how immigrants are handled; public health needs to be as important as acute care; partnerships are important; and public trust needs to be developed and maintained (Interlandi, 2023). States struggled as they entered the pandemic with long-term budget cuts, staffing shortages, inadequate technology, and many other problems, such as coping with the many residents who lacked adequate health insurance. They were not ready to cope with a significant public health emergency and collaborate and coordinate with other states and the federal government.

The Federal Emergency Management Agency (FEMA) has developed the *Guides to Expanding Mitigation*, which are part of a series that supports innovative and emerging partnerships for **mitigation**, or actions taken to reduce the seriousness of an event or a problem. This information is provided to assist communities in better supporting hazard mitigation projects and planning by engaging other sectors and building partnerships. The purpose is to support FEMA's goal of building a culture of preparedness, which is part of the agency's strategic plan (FEMA, 2022). Public health emergency mitigation planning needs to consider collaboration with the following stakeholders and other health-related groups (FEMA, 2022):

- Senior care organizations and extended care organizations
- Faith-based organizations
- Community-based organizations
- Public housing agencies or authorities
- Dialysis centers
- Community health centers
- Hospitals
- First responders
- Health emergency preparedness coalitions
- Public health and emergency preparedness coordinators
- Federal, state, and local health departments and agencies
- Academic institutions
- Community schools
- Public transportation authorities
- Community businesses

Mitigation should focus on (FEMA, 2022):

- Collaboration between emergency managers, community planners, and public health officials can lead to:
- Identifying toxic sites within the floodplain or near potable and well water sources
- Sharing insight into how vulnerability to hazards varies across populations and the ways in which children, older adults, low-income communities, public housing residents, and some communities may be disproportionately affected
- Identifying resiliency or preparedness investments that address the unique vulnerabilities across these populations
- Identifying health services and mental health providers that are not listed as critical facilities
- Identifying critical records stored in hazardous areas that should be relocated and digitized
- Combining risk awareness and emergency preparedness campaigns with existing public health campaigns and engaging with health officials as part of their planning process

Local, state, and federal governments develop and implement policies to ensure public health and safety during community emergencies; they also influence clinical practice. As noted with the crisis standards, "public health emergencies require clinicians to change their practice, including, in some situations, acting to prioritize the community above the individual in fairly allocating scarce resources" (Berlinger et al., 2020).

Public Health Nursing and Policy

Nurses have an important responsibility in participating in health policy development, implementation, and evaluation (Anders, 2021). Nurses participate in clinical practice, research, and academic settings and serve as advocates, and health policies affect all these activities. Nurses have expertise that can add to the policymaking process, but they also need to be aware of policies and their implications to health care, nursing practice, and the profession. This requires keeping up to date with policies, even before they are developed and implemented. An example of the need to be aware is when the COVID-19 pandemic required changes in existing policies and the development of new guidelines. Nurses advocated for many of these policies to protect the public and healthcare workers, such as mitigation interventions (e.g., masking, personal protective equipment, testing, vaccinations, limiting large crowds). Nurses who hold staff positions in government or may be elected officials can participate directly in the policy process in both cases. As has been noted in this content, it is important for nurses to be prepared in health policy—understanding the process, roles and responsibilities, and outcomes. Nursing education must include this content in all levels of nursing education programs.

Healthy People 2030 and Other Major Government Initiatives: Impact on Health Policy

Healthy People 2030 is a major national public health initiative managed by the HHS that provides a comprehensive plan focused on health promotion and disease prevention. It identifies goals and objectives that are used to routinely assesses national health status. **Appendix B** provides an overview of this initiative. The goals include an aim directly related to policy—use health policy to prevent disease and improve health—and identify the following as important:

> Health policy can have a major impact on health and well-being. Healthy People 2030 focuses on keeping people safe and healthy through laws and policies at the local, state, territorial, and federal level. Evidence-based health policies can help prevent disease and promote health. For example, smoke-free policies can help prevent smoking initiation and increase quit attempts. Similarly, policies requiring community water systems to provide fluoridated water can improve oral health. Establishing informed policies is key to improving health nationwide. (ODPHP, 2020)

Another major federal initiative is the NHQDR. For 19 years, the HHS, through the AHRQ, has managed a monitoring system to assess and provide data about healthcare quality and disparity. The AHRQ provides an annual report to monitor the U.S. system and health status and publishes an annual report of heath quality and disparities. Originally, the policy guiding this initiative provided two reports, one on quality and another on health disparities. It was then decided that the two issues were critical to one another and that one report would be more effective. The monitoring process used for the analysis includes measures focused on access to care, affordable care, care coordination, effective treatment, healthy living, patient safety, and person-centered care (AHRQ, 2022c).

Examine the objectives associated with the Healthy People 2030 policy goal.

Website: https://health.gov/healthypeople/objectives-and-data/browse-objectives/health-policy

Quality Improvement

Quality improvement (QI) is an important health policy issue. It focuses on access, quality and safety, and outcomes. Historically, most QI has been more concerned with acute health care; however, it is also important in regard to public health. It is more difficult to monitor and intervene in public health due to the multiple services, settings, healthcare providers, and stakeholders as well as governmental influence. Public health QI must also consider issues related to population health, whereas acute care QI focuses more on individuals. There is no single agency or organization that is responsible for overall population health improvement, although the HHS and its agencies have assumed much of this responsibility and local and state health departments should be actively engaged, which requires collaboration and coordination. Public polices need to support effective QI. The goal is to improve the health of every person and population in their communities through planning and coordinating to ensure measurement, innovation, collaboration, and improvement to achieve the Triple Aim goals of better care, smarter spending, and healthier people and communities (CMS, 2021).

The CDC implemented the National Public Health Improvement Initiative (NPHII) to assist 73 public health agencies in increasing public health accreditation readiness, improving efficiency and effectiveness through QI initiatives, and increasing performance management capacity. Through the NPHII, agencies increased their ability to make data-driven decisions for priority setting, program planning, and implementation; eliminated siloes through partnerships and collaborations; strengthened the culture for performance improvement; and institutionalized these practices within the agency.

Examples of Health Problems With Major Public Health Implications

The following are some of the current health problems that have major public health implications and require consideration in public policymaking at the local, state, and federal levels as well as by private healthcare organizations:

- **Mental health:** An increasing number of people of all ages are experiencing mental health problems. Some of this rise is due to the stress from COVID-19 as a health issue and the methods used to prevent the illness (e.g., reducing social activities, loss of work, limited family time, using digital methods for work and school, masking). Policies related to assessing needs and providing services in communities, workplace, and schools need to consider the best methods and costs.

This also requires qualified healthcare providers, which relates to funding for healthcare professional programs and the consideration of relevant content and experiences to prepare providers, as seen in earlier examples about funding for workforce development.

- **Violence:** Violence in communities of all types (rural, urban, and many settings [e.g., workplace, schools, public areas]) has increased and affects all ages. Losing a family member or friend through violence does not go away; rather, it leads to long-term feelings of loss. Fear, anxiety, and depression can be experienced by individuals, families, and communities after a violent event.
- **Opioid epidemic:** The use of opioids has been increasing for many years. For some communities, it is at the crisis point—an epidemic. This problem affects health in general and can lead to death. It is a complex problem that must be assessed and addressed. Substance use disorders are lifetime disorders.

For these types of public health problems, policymaking needs to consider the assessment of needs; the provision of services in communities, workplace, and schools; as well as the most appropriate prevention and intervention methods and costs. This also requires qualified healthcare providers, which relates to funding for healthcare professional programs and consideration of relevant content and experiences to prepare providers. These health issues are also examples of problems that are related to the SDOH and that require engagement from other areas, such as social services, law enforcement, and the legal system. This is complex, and there is disagreement as to the best approaches to reduce these health problems. As public health issues, they affect activities throughout a community and can lead to long-term challenges and death (e.g., shootings, suicide, and automobile accidents). Every community should assess its level of need and take steps to reduce these issues. This may require policies and laws related to gun control, drug surveillance and actions, transportation safety, and other measures. These issues need to be addressed not only by government policies but also in the private sector. This is recognized by major organizations such as the IHI, which offered a workshop on the role of health systems in gun violence focusing on collaboration between major stakeholders and communication (IHI, 2023b). The workshop speakers were experts in healthcare quality and other issues experienced by healthcare providers. This is an important discussion as many consider gun violence to be an epidemic that affects the public at all levels and that has aroused conflict as to the most appropriate policies to reduce this problem.

Drugs and Approvals: Implications for Public Health Policy

A recent problem that is increasing that has policy implications is drug shortages (Jewett, 2023). Some common reasons for these shortages, which are global, include manufacturing and quality problems, misapplication of FDA approval and inspection procedures, and discontinuation of drugs. The shortages have serious implications for health and public trust in the health system. The government at the federal level is involved in responding to this problem. For example, the U.S. Senate Committee on Homeland Security and Governmental Affairs (HSGAC) issued a report that identified the following as key issues related to drug shortages, and these affect current policies and the need for changes or new guidelines (HSGAC, 2023):

1. Drug shortages are increasing, lasting longer, and affecting patient care.
2. Overreliance on foreign and geographically concentrated sources for critical drugs and their key starting materials and limited domestic manufacturing capabilities create health and national security risks.
3. The FDA still lacks critical information that could help mitigate shortages.
4. While the FDA retains certain data from manufacturers on the pharmaceutical supply chain, such as key starting materials needed to make drug substances, those data are currently not provided or stored in a useable format to aid supply chain visibility.
5. Industry and the federal government lack end-to-end visibility into the pharmaceutical supply chain, and efforts to map supply chains are not sufficiently coordinated.
6. The FDA lacks authority to require manufacturer recalls for most drug products.

The AMA is also concerned about these shortages. It adopted a policy that emphasized that the drug shortages are a public health crisis (AMA, 2020). This is an example of how a private healthcare professional organization can actively enter policymaking and offer its expertise. The AMA recommends that changes be made to mitigate drug shortages, such as those specifically related to manufacturing innovations, global supply chain transparency, and drug maker incentives. Policy changes are required to collaborate with stakeholders, including the drug industry, and reduce the problem to ensure patients can receive the drugs they need when they need them.

Refugee, Immigrant, and Migrant Workers

The presence of refugee, immigrant, and migrant workers (RIM) has an impact on public health needs in many communities. The HHS and its agencies such as the CDC work "with partners to connect mobile populations with domestic resources to ensure a continuum of care that helps them live healthy, active, and productive lives in their new communities" (CDC, 2022d). To meet these needs, many stakeholders are involved, such as community- and faith-based organizations, employers, healthcare systems and providers, public health agencies, policymakers, and others such as federal government agencies (e.g., the Department of State, Immigration and Customs Enforcement, U.S. Citizenship and Immigration Services, and the Department of Homeland Security). The goals are to promote fair access to health (i.e., equity) and improve opportunity. RIM public health needs are directly associated with the SDOH and with public policy that addresses these issues. Diversity and language are critical elements that must be considered to ensure health equity and literacy as well as effective health services within these communities.

Technology and Digital Health

Policy is an important factor in the development and use of technology, both for healthcare professionals' use and for personal use. Social media has expanded and is now part of the daily lives of many Americans. In one review, it was noted that 5.03 billion individuals use the Internet globally, and 59% of this population uses social media (Kemp, 2022). Technology can be used by all stakeholders, either formally, such as a healthcare organization providing health information to its communities, or informally, such as individuals sharing information. For example, during the COVID-19 pandemic, nurses used social media to advocate for policies to protect the public and themselves, providing a method for voices to actively participate with limited barriers (Anders, 2021). However, nurses should use social media carefully, sharing accurate and timely information and supporting the nursing code of ethics (ANA, 2015).

Digital health (telehealth and telemedicine) has increased, and there is no doubt that COVID-19 has been a driving force in this expansion, which required changes in policies and new guidelines from the government level and private sector. This process will continue as digital health outcomes are evaluated and new methods are used. One new method that will need extensive policy consideration to ensure the public's safety and positive health outcomes is the development of **artificial intelligence** (AI), which uses computer and technology science to make decisions that might be made by human intelligence. It is not known what the impact of AI might have in the long term on health care, but the HHS recognizes this as an area that needs to be addressed (e.g., AI information is included in the HHS website [HHS, 2023g]). The HHS response includes assigning staff and leadership to AI and identifying an AI strategy for HHS:

> Set forth an approach and focus areas intended to encourage AI adoption; enable HHS-wide familiarity, comfort, and fluency with artificial intelligence (AI) technology and its potential; promote AI scaling with the application of best practices and lessons learned from piloting and implementing AI capabilities to additional domains and use cases across HHS; and spark AI acceleration by increasing the speed at which HHS adopts and scales AI and ML [machine learning]. (HHS, 2023g)

The HHS also identifies statutes or laws associated with this new area that require active policy development and the consideration of such issues as research, health services, regulations, funding, and evaluation. As AI is developed and implemented, more policies will need to be expanded to address any problems and ensure the quality of care, equity, and privacy and security of information.

The Pew Research Center reported that 72% of Americans use social media for health reasons, such as obtaining health information and for support (2023). What does this mean for health policy? Technology is an area connected to policy that guides what can be done with technology, reimbursement (e.g., for digital health), and regulations regarding technology, among other issues. Since social media is actively used by the public, anything that affects it then makes a difference in public use and reliability of information. Whether information comes from a credible source is a critical question. As was noted during the COVID-19 pandemic, misinformation and disinformation were serious problems, and social media drove the sharing of much of this information. An example of policy's effect on this issue at the state level is the legislation approved in California that instituted punishment for physicians who spread false information about COVID-19 vaccination and treatment that then had an impact on public health (Myers, 2023; 2022). In this case, what is the difference between a law and a policy? A law was passed in California that identifies this action as professional misconduct, and since it is now a law, it has legal implications. States are responsible for the licensure and regulations related to healthcare practice, and they make and implement policies related to practice. In January 2023, a federal court temporarily blocked the enforcement of this new law, which was the first U.S. law to address medical misinformation during a time of public health crisis. The resolution of this legal case as well as another associated case will take time.

Search the Internet to find any updates on this new law and legal concerns. Key terms you might use include *California law of doctor misinformation* and *COVID-19 professional misconduct law California.*

What is the status of the legal case? Why are this law and then the follow-up legal action important to public health and public health emergencies?

The federal government has taken steps to make providing and receiving care through telehealth and digital health easier (HHS, 2023h). Examples of policy areas the HHS identifies as important are HIPAA and telehealth technology, Medicare and Medicaid policies, provider licensure, prescription of controlled substances, remote patient monitoring, and policy changes during COVID-19. As part of its policymaking, the HHS 2020–2025 Federal Health IT Strategic Plan identifies key principles, as shown in **Figure 9.**

Put individuals first.
Embrace person-centered care that values the whole individual, including their goals, values, culture, and privacy.
Focus on value.
Promote and pursue activities that improve health and care quality, efficiency, safety, affordability, equity, effectiveness, and access.
Build a culture of secure access to health information.
Support secure health information access, exchange, and use by individuals, caregivers, healthcare providers, public health professionals, and other stakeholders.
Put research into action.
Strengthen feedback loops between scientific, public health, and healthcare communities to efficiently translate evidence into clinical practice and improvement.
Encourage innovation and competition.
Support and protect innovation and competition in health IT that result in new solutions and business models for better care and improved outcomes.
Be a responsible steward.
Develop health IT policies through open, transparent, and accountable processes; use federal resources judiciously; and leverage the expertise of the private sector to provide technology and services to execute on these policies, as appropriate.

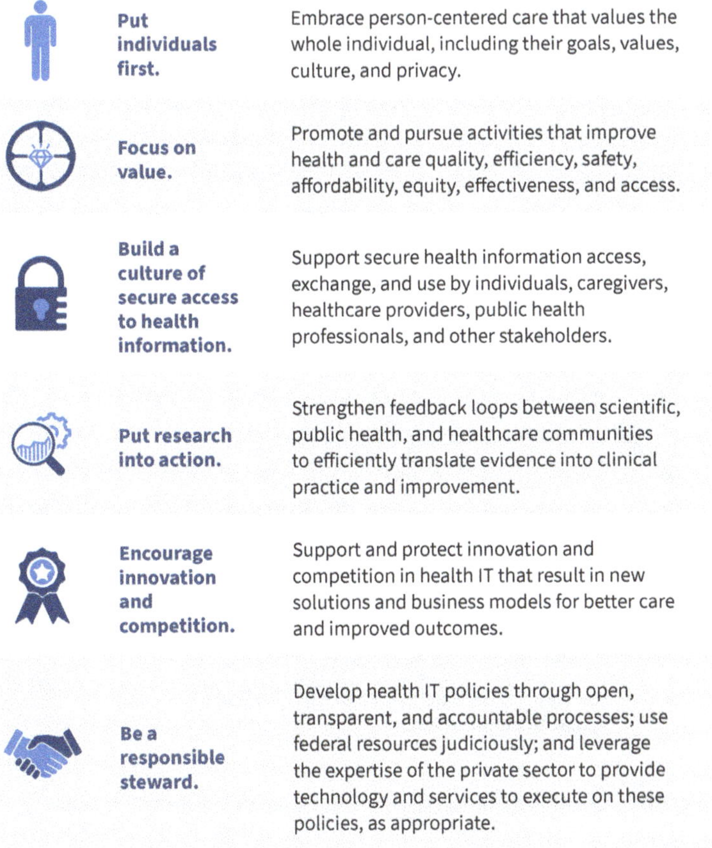

Figure 9. 2020–2025 Federal Health IT Strategic Plan

Rural Health and Public Policy

Rural communities experience many public health challenges (HRSA, 2019). Workforce issues are a problem in these areas and are associated with barriers to cross-state licensure. This is a policy issue in that any changes made to licensure regulations could have a positive impact on the workforce shortage. One type of policy change is the option to use interstate compact licensure for registered nurses, which allows nurses to have a license in one state and practice in a nearby one, if the states have agreed legally to this arrangement (i.e., established a policy approving it). Another example of a change in policy that occurred during the COVID-19 pandemic that increased access to services and reduced the problem of state-based licensure is the CARES Act (Cram, 2023). This law allowed CMS reimbursement for telehealth services that did not require providers to be in the same state as their patients. Both examples of licensure issues are policies that have assisted public health in rural communities. **Figure 10** describes some issues related to rural health care, coordination, and collaboration that affect policies.

Safety net healthcare providers are providers that provide a significant amount of health care to patients with limited or no insurance coverage. Many of these services are found in rural communities (see **Exhibit 4**), and they face a unique combination of challenges, including limited economies of scale, heavy dependence on public payers, low patient volume, and unnecessary duplication

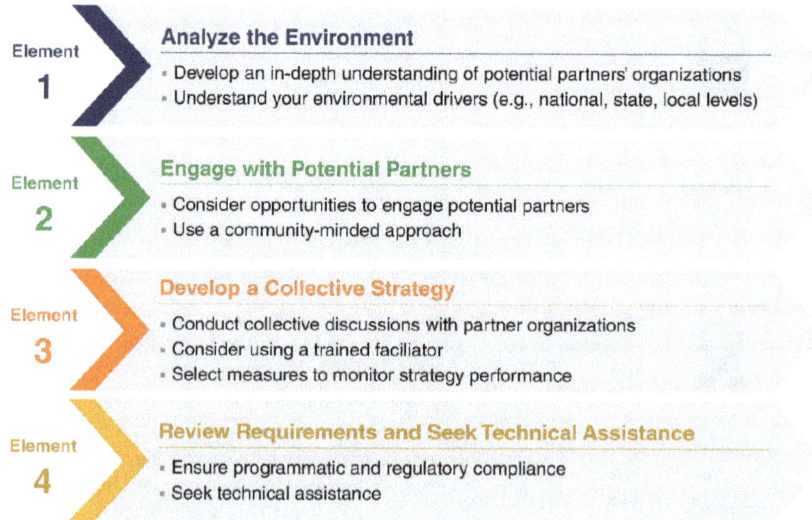

Figure 10. Rural Health Care Collaboration and Coordination: Areas of Consideration

of services among providers. Given these circumstances, rural providers such as the health centers/federally qualified health centers (CMS program/policy), small rural hospitals (local and state policies, laws, accreditation, and CMS), critical access hospitals (Balanced Budget Act of 1997, Public Law 105-33; Medicare Rural Hospital Flexibility Program), rural health clinics (CMS), and local public health departments (local and state health policies and laws) may compete for limited resources, staff, and patients in their communities. These programs are guided by public policies, as noted in **Exhibit** 4.

Exhibit 4: Key Lessons and Rural Health

Key Lessons Learned from Rural Health Leaders on Implementing Collaboration and Coordination Strategies

1. Leverage use of existing data sources to inform meaningful collaboration and coordination
- Organizations can use existing information, such as needs assessments and electronic health record (EHR) data, to identify the needs of the patient population and the organizations that can best meet those needs.
- Reviewing public information sources (e.g., strategic plans, regulatory filings, needs assessments, and technical reports) can help deepen the understanding of other organizations in the community and identify shared priorities.

2. Engage potential partners
- The community health needs assessment process can be an opportunity to engage with potential partners.
- Organizations with no prior history of collaboration might start with a small-scale project to establish a working relationship for larger projects.
- Taking a "community-minded" approach can encourage engagement with other potential partner organizations, recognizing that no single organization can address all of the community's needs.

3. Develop a collective strategy
- Collaborations are more effective when designed collectively by all participating organizations, rather than being initiated and dominated by a single organization.

4. Commit to transparency and honest communication
- Candid and honest conversations among potential partner organizations can result in clear expectations and role delineations.
- When a relationship between two organizations has a strong foundation of trust, sharing board members can be an effective way to increase transparency and enhance collaboration/coordination.

5. Set realistic expectations and prepare for potential changes
- Not every strategy will be successful; failed strategies and partnerships can provide valuable learning experiences that enhance the success of future partnerships.
- Leaders are important to establishing and maintaining collaboration and coordination; however, leaders will likely change. Formally document partnerships through memoranda of agreement (MOA) or memoranda of understanding (MOU) so that collaboration and coordination efforts can survive the departure of the leaders who initiated them.

6. Identify measures to monitor progress and performance
- Identifying meaningful measures helps guide improvement and performance of collaboration/coordination efforts.
- Use of performance measures data can help garner sustainability support from others in the community.

7. Complete due diligence before committing to a strategy
- All organizations involved in a collaboration/coordination strategy must first ensure that the strategy complies with all of their programmatic and regulatory requirements.

Source: U.S. Department of Health and Human Services, Health Resources and Services Administration. (2019). A guide for rural health care collaboration. *https://www.hrsa.gov/sites/default/files/hrsa/rural-health/resources/hrsa-rural-collaboration-guide.pdf*

The CFC has discussed the need for improvement within the public health system, which requires a more effective coordinated system to protect public health and respond to health emergencies. This is a private organization, and yet it is engaged in both private and public policy development. The CFC assessment provides a solid summary point about public policy and improvement and identifies the following principles that should be used by U.S. Congress; the Biden-Harris administration; and states, localities, tribes, and territories to offer policy for public health improvement (CFC, 2022b):

- The federal government should lead a strong and capable national public health system.
- Congress should provide stable support matched with clear expectations for states, localities, tribes, and territories to protect the health of their populations.

- The healthcare system should work closely with public health agencies in normal times and during emergencies.
- The public health system should earn the public's trust.

Summary

This content examined the relationship between healthcare delivery, public policy, and public and community health. Both public and private policies are integral to the public's health. Important factors that should be considered when examining health policies and policymaking are DEIA and the SDOH, both of which influence public and community health. Policy development must consider content and an effective process to arrive at a policy as well as its implementation and evaluation. The legislative process is important, as is the role of government at all levels (local, stage, national, and even global). Funding is related to policies and is needed to develop and then implement and evaluate them, and reimbursement may be a factor if a policy relates to providing services. Along with funding issues, policymakers need to use the best evidence to support policy content and implementation. As noted in this content, there are many issues that require policy consideration, such as public health emergencies, public health nursing, drugs and approval, telehealth, and rural health, among others discussed.

Discussion Questions

1. Why is public policy relevant to public and community health?
2. How does DEIA relate to public policy?
3. What are the key components in the public policy process?
4. How are research and evidence-informed public health policy related?
5. Why should healthcare providers be involved in health policy?

References

Act for Public Health. (2023). *Support and resources for strengthening public health protections.* https://actforpublichealth.org/

Agency for Healthcare Research and Quality. (2022a). *Consumer Assessment of Healthcare Providers and Systems (CAHPS®) 2022 virtual research meeting summary: Assessing patient experience for insights into enhancing equity in healthcare*. U.S. Department of Health and Human Services. https://www.ahrq.gov/sites/default/files/wysiwyg/cahps/news-and-events/events/webinars/cahps-virtual-research-meeting-summary_2022.pdf

Agency for Healthcare Research and Quality. (2022b). *Six domains of healthcare quality*. U.S. Department of Health and Human Services. https://www.ahrq.gov/talkingquality/measures/six-domains.html

Agency for Healthcare Quality and Research. (2022c). *National Healthcare Quality and Disparities Reports*. U.S. Department of Health and Human Services https://www.ahrq.gov/research/findings/nhqrdr/index.html

Agency for Healthcare Research and Quality. (2023a). *Center for Evidence and Practice Improvement (CEPI)*. U.S. Department of Health and Human Services. https://www.ahrq.gov/cpi/centers/cepi/index.html

Agency for Healthcare Research and Quality. (2023b). *About AHRQ*. U.S. Department of Health and Human Services. https://www.ahrq.gov/cpi/about/index.html

American Association of Colleges of Nursing. (2021). *The essentials: Core competencies for professional nursing education*. https://www.aacnnursing.org/essentials

American Association of Colleges of Nursing. (2023). *Federal policy agenda*. https://www.aacnnursing.org/policy-advocacy/federal-policy-agenda

American Hospital Association. (2020). *Pathways to population health*. https://www.aha.org/system/files/media/file/2020/09/Pathways-to-Population-Health-Framework.pdf

American Hospital Association. (2023a). *AHA comments on reauthorization of the Pandemic and All-Hazards Preparedness Act (PAHPA)*. https://www.aha.org/lettercomment/2023-03-29-aha-comments-reauthorization-pandemic-and-all-hazards-preparedness-act-pahpa

American Hospital Association. (2023b). *About the AHA*. https://www.aha.org/about

American Medical Association. (2020). *AMA strengthens policy to combat spike in national drug shortages*. https://www.ama-assn.org/press-center/press-releases/ama-strengthens-policy-combat-spike-national-drug-shortages

American Nurses Association. (2015). *Code of ethics for nurses*. https://www.nursingworld.org/practice-policy/nursing-excellence/ethics/code-of-ethics-for-nurses/

American Nurses Association. (2018). *ANA political action committee*. https://ana.aristotle.com/SitePages/pac.aspx

American Nurses Association. (2023a). *Health policies*. https://www.nursingworld.org/practice-policy/health-policy/

American Nurses Association. (2023b). *Federal advocacy*. https://www.nursingworld.org/practice-policy/advocacy/federal/

American Nurses Association. (2023c). *Minority fellowship program*. https://www.nursingworld.org/practice-policy/workforce/minority-fellowship-program/

American Nurses Association. (2023d). *Washington policy fellowship program*. https://www.nursingworld.org/foundation/programs/washington-policy-fellowship/

American Organization for Nursing Leadership. (2023). *Key issues for nurses.* https://www.aonl.org/advocacy/key-issues

American Public Health Association. (2021). *Creating the healthiest nation: Advancing health equity.* https://www.apha.org/-/media/files/pdf/factsheets/advancing_health_equity.ashx

American Public Health Association. (2022). *Generation public health.* https://www.apha.org/what-is-public-health/generation-public-health

American Public Health Association. (2023a). *Centering and celebrating cultures in health toolkit.* https://nphw.org/Tools-and-Tips/Toolkit

American Public Health Association. (2023b). *Action alerts.* https://apha.org/policies-and-advocacy/advocacy-for-public-health/action-alerts

Anders, R. (2021). Engaging nurses in health policy in the era of COVID-19. *Nursing Forum, 56*(1), 89–94.

Benadjaoud, Y., & Romero, L. (2023). *States warn of health care worker shortage as they prep for next pandemic.* ABC News. https://abcnews.go.com/Health/states-warn-health-care-worker-shortage-prep-pandemic/story?id=98160609

Berlinger, N., Wynia, M., Powell, T., et al. (2020). *Ethical framework for health care institutions & guidelines for institutional ethics services responding to the coronavirus pandemic.* Hastings Center, March 16. 2020. https://www.thehastingscenter.org/ethicalframeworkcovid-19/

Bhattacharya, D., & Bhatt, J. (2017). Seven foundational principles of population health policy. *Population Health Management, 20*(5), 383–388. https://repository.usfca.edu/cgi/viewcontent.cgi?article=1131&context=nursing_fac

Brownson, R., Seiler, R., & Eyeler, A. (2010). Measuring the impact of public health policy. *Prevention Chronic Disease, 7*(4), A77. http://www.cdc.gov/pcd/issues/2010/jul/09_0249.htm

Centers for Disease Control and Prevention. (2016). *Health in all policies.* U.S. Department of Health and Human Services. https://www.cdc.gov/policy/hiap/index.html

Centers for Disease Control and Prevention. (2020). *What is population health?* U.S. Department of Health and Human Services. https://www.cdc.gov/pophealthtraining/whatis.html

Centers for Disease Control and Prevention. (2021a). *What is health literacy?* U.S. Department of Health and Human Services. https://www.cdc.gov/healthliteracy/learn/

Centers for Disease Control and Prevention. (2021b). *The CDC policy process.* U.S. Department of Health and Human Services. https://www.cdc.gov/policy/polaris/training/policy-process/index.html

Centers for Disease Control and Prevention. (2021c). *Health policy brief.* U.S. Department of Health and Human Services. https://www.cdc.gov/policy/polaris/training/writing-briefs/index.html

Centers for Disease Control and Prevention. (2022a). *Mission, role, and pledge.* U.S. Department of Health and Human Services. https://www.cdc.gov/about/organization/mission.htm

Centers for Disease Control and Prevention. (2022b). *Social determinants of health*. U.S. Department of Health and Human Services. U.S. Department of Health and Human Services. https://www.cdc.gov/about/sdoh/index.html

Centers for Disease Control and Prevention. (2022c). *National health initiatives, strategies, and action plans*. U.S. Department of Health and Human Services. https://www.cdc.gov/publichealthgateway/strategy/index.html

Centers for Disease Control and Prevention. (2022d). *Immigrant, refugee, and migrant health*. U.S. Department of Health and Human Services. https://www.cdc.gov/immigrantrefugeehealth/about-irmh.html

Centers for Disease Control and Prevention. (2023a). *About us*. U.S. Department of Health and Human Services. https://www.cdc.gov/phlp/about/index.html

Centers for Disease Control and Prevention. (2023a). *What is health equity?* U.S. Department of Health and Human Services. https://www.cdc.gov/nchhstp/healthequity/index.html

Centers for Disease Control and Prevention. (2023b). *Laws and regulations*. U.S. Department of Health and Human Services. https://www.hhs.gov/regulations/index.html

Centers for Disease Control and Prevention, Division of Population Health. (2021). *Population health*. U.S. Department of Health and Human Services. https://www.cdc.gov/populationhealth/index.html

Centers for Medicare & Medicaid Services. (2021). *Population health measures*. U.S. Department of Health and Human Services. https://mmshub.cms.gov/sites/default/files/Population-Health-Measures.pdf

Centers for Medicare & Medicaid Services. (2023a). *End of the federal COVID-19 public health emergency (PHE) declaration*. U.S. Department of Health and Human Services. https://www.cdc.gov/coronavirus/2019-ncov/your-health/end-of-phe.html

Centers for Medicare & Medicaid Services. (2023b). *Accountable health communities model*. U.S. Department of Health and Human Services. https://innovation.cms.gov/innovation-models/ahcm

Center for Strategic and International Studies. (2023). *Building the CDC the country needs*. https://www.csis.org/analysis/building-cdc-country-needs

Chappel, A., et al. (2022). Improving health and well-being through community care hubs. *Health Affairs Forefront. https://www.healthaffairs.org/content/forefront/improving-health-and-well-being-through-community-care-hubs*

Chase, R. (2023). *University of Delaware agrees to settle class-action case over COVID campus shutdown*. ABC News. https://apnews.com/article/covid-university-delaware-lawsuit-settlement-d2b647ee1923d79cd011b1ac6fddd3d2

Cohen, R., & Cha, A. (2022). *Health insurance coverage: Early release of estimates from the national health interview survey, 2022*. https://www.cdc.gov/nchs/data/nhis/earlyrelease/insur202305_1.pdf

Collins, K., & Luhby, T. (2022). *COVID-19 remains a public health emergency in the U.S., administration says*. CNN. https://edition.cnn.com/2022/05/17/politics/covid-19-public-health-emergency/index.html

Commonwealth Fund Commission. (2022a). *Meeting America's public health challenge.* https://www.commonwealthfund.org/publications/fund-reports/2022/jun/meeting-americas-public-health-challenge

Commonwealth Fund Commission. (2022b). *Nonpartisan commission of health leaders calls for building a national public health system.* https://www.commonwealthfund.org/press-release/2022/nonpartisan-commission-health-leaders-calls-building-national-public-health

Commonwealth Fund. (2023). *About us.* https://www.commonwealthfund.org/about-us

Congress.gov. (2022). *S.674—Public Health Infrastructure Saves Lives Act.* https://www.congress.gov/bill/117th-congress/senate-bill/674

Conyers-Tucker, H., Brou, L., & Goldbert, D. (2022). Structural stigma in law: Implications and opportunities for health and health equity. *Health Affairs.* December 8, 2022. https://www.healthaffairs.org/do/10.1377/hpb20221104.659710/full/?utm_medium=email&utm_source=hasu&utm_campaign=HASU+12+11+2022&utm_content=policy+brief&utm_term=structural+stigma+in+law&vgo_ee=JtfE9pVmuWUZhGM0zRZvGAA3SuMkJhmkGexv49sZvNU%3D`

Council on Linkages Between Academia and Public Health Practice. (2021). *Core competencies for public health professionals.* http://www.phf.org/resourcestools/pages/core_public_health_competencies.aspx

Cram, A. (2023). *Telehealth and licensure policies improving healthcare access for rural communities.* https://www.astho.org/communications/blog/telehealth-licensure-policies-improving-access-for-rural-communities/?utm_campaign=enews20230216&utm_medium=email&utm_source=govdelivery

Cubanski, J., Kates, J., Tolbert, J., et al. (2023). *What happens when COVID-19 emergency declarations end? Implications for coverage, costs, and access.* KFF. https://www.kff.org/coronavirus-covid-19/issue-brief/what-happens-when-covid-19-emergency-declarations-end-implications-for-coverage-costs-and-access/

D'Lima, D., Soukup, T., & Hull, L. (2021). Evaluating the application of the RE-AIM planning and evaluation framework: An updated systematic review and exploration of pragmatic application. *Frontiers in Public Health, 9.* https://www.ncbi.nlm.nih.gov/pmc/articles/PMC8826088/Federal

Federal Emergency Management Administration. (2022). *FEMA strategic plan 2022-2026.* https://www.fema.gov/about/strategic-plan

Federal Register. (2021). *Advancing racial equity and support for underserved communities through the federal government. Executive Order 13985.* January 20, 2021. https://www.federalregister.gov/documents/2021/01/25/2021-01753/advancing-racial-equity-and-support-for-underserved-communities-through-the-federal-government

Finkelman, A. (2023a). *Health equity and disparities.* Cognella, Inc.

Finkelman, A. (2023b). *Population health and vulnerable populations.* Cognella, Inc.

Glasgow, R. E., Harden, S. M., Gaglio, B., et al. (2019). RE-AIM planning and evaluation framework: Adapting to new science and practice with a 20-year review. *Frontiers in Public Health*, *7* (March). https://doi.org/10.3389/fpubh.2019.00064

Health Resources and Services Administration. (2019). *A guide for rural healthcare collaboration and coordination*. U.S. Department of Health and Human Services. https://www.hrsa.gov/sites/default/files/hrsa/rural-health/resources/hrsa-rural-collaboration-guide.pdf

Health Resources and Services Administration. (2023a). *About HRSA*. U.S. Department of Health and Human Services. https://www.hrsa.gov/about

Health Resources and Services Administration. (2023b). *HRSA joins HHS partners to support states and other partners' work during the unwinding of the COVID-19 public health emergency and continuous Medicaid enrollment*. U.S. Department of Health and Human Services. https://www.hrsa.gov/about/news/press-releases/april-2023-roundup

Health Resources and Services Administration. (2023c). *Nurse Education, Practice, Quality and Retention (NEPQR) Simulation Education Training (SET) program*. U.S. Department of Health and Human Services. https://www.hrsa.gov/grants/find-funding/HRSA-23-129?utm_campaign=enews20230615&utm_medium=email&utm_source=govdelivery

Health Resources and Services Administration. (2023d). *Medicaid unwinding and returning to regular operations after COVID-19*. U.S. Department of Health and Human Services. https://www.hrsa.gov/about/news/press-releases/phe-transition?utm_campaign=enews20230518&utm_medium=email&utm_source=govdelivery

Hick, J., Hanfling, D., Wynia, M. K., & Toner, E. (2021). Crisis standards of care and COVID-19: What did we learn? How do we ensure equity? What should we do? *NAM Perspectives*. https://doi.org/10.31478%2F202108e

Inglesby, T., & Morrison, J. (2023, May 7). How to overhaul the CDC. *The New York Times*. https://www.nytimes.com/2023/05/07/opinion/cdc-overhaul.html

Institute for Healthcare Improvement. (2023a). *IHI triple aim improvement*. https://www.ihi.org/Engage/Initiatives/TripleAim/Pages/default.aspx

Institute for Healthcare Improvement. (2023b). *Role of health systems in gun violence*. https://www.ihi.org/education/Conferences/National-Forum/Pages/roundtable.aspx?utm_campaign=23%20Forum&utm_medium=email&_hsmi=262358423&_hsenc=p2ANqtz-9DIGRSa5jzK7eFUZ63QRWSyroqD8AIpMcSzfAts05FCkDG7v6aO9YwuuZVV21JjYodorh25wZ1pHJGJa_Gj9sIyIULDA&utm_content=262358423&utm_source=hs_email

Institute of Medicine. (2012). *Crises standards of care: A systems framework for catastrophic disaster response*. The National Academies Press.

Interlandi, J. (2020). Why we're losing the battle with COVID-19. *The New York Times*, July 14, 2020. https://www.nytimes.com/2020/07/14/magazine/covid-19-public-health-texas.html

Interlandi, J. (2023). American is forgetting the lessons of COVID health emergency. *The New York Times*, May 11, 2023. https://www.nytimes.com/2023/05/11/opinion/covid-pandemic-emergency-lessons.html

Jewett, C. (2023). Drug shortages near all-time high, leading to rationing. *The New York Times*, May 17, 2023. https://www.nytimes.com/2023/05/17/health/drug-shortages-cancer.html

Johnston, L., & Finegood, D. (2015). Opportunities for addressing obesity and noncommunicable disease through engagement with the private sector. *Annual Review of Public Health, 36*, 255–271. https://doi.org/10.1146/annurev-publhealth-031914-122802

Jolley, C., & Peck, J. (2022). Diversity, equity, & inclusion policies in national nursing organizations. *OJIN: The Online Journal of Nursing, 27*(2), Manuscript 2. https://www.doi.org/10.3912/OJIN.Vol27No02Man02

Kemp, S. (2022). *Digital 2022: July global Statshot report*. DataReportal, July 21, 2022. https://datareportal.com/reports/digital-2022-july-global-statshot

Kiff, L. (2023). Obamacare mandate for preventive care is restored, for now. *The New York Times*, June 23, 2023. https://www.nytimes.com/2023/06/12/health/obamacare-preventive-care.html

Kindig, D., & Stoddart G. (2003). What is population health? *American Journal of Public Health, 93*(3), 380–383.

Krueger, J. (2023). *Act for public health: Assessing legislation and litigation impacting public health authority*. Network for Public Health Law, January 26, 2023. https://www.networkforphl.org/resources/act-for-public-health-assessing-legislation-and-litigation-impacting-public-health-authority

LaVeist, T. A., Pérez-Stable, E. J., Richard, P., et al. (2023). The economic burden of racial, ethnic, and educational health inequities in the US. *JAMA, 329*(19), 1682–1692.

Mahr, K. (2022). *CDC director orders agency overhaul, admitting flawed Covid-19 response*. Politico. https://www.politico.com/news/2022/08/17/cdc-agency-overhaul-covid-19-response-00052384

Mittmann, H., Heinrich, J., & Levi, J. (2022). Accountable communities for health: What we are learning from recent evaluations. *NAM Perspectives*. Discussion paper, National Academy of Medicine. https://nam.edu/accountable-communities-for-health-what-we-are-learning-from-recent-evaluations/

Morrison, J. S., & Inglesby, T. (2023). *Building the CDC the country needs*. https://csis-website-prod.s3.amazonaws.com/s3fs-public/publication/230112_Morrison_Building_CDC.pdf?VersionId=kTKB3urWn1bfZpXuCqixfxzHfT8AUcIM

Myers, S. (2022). California approves bill to punish doctors who spread false information. *The New York Times*, August 29, 2022. https://www.nytimes.com/2022/08/29/technology/california-doctors-covid-misinformation.html

Myers, S. (2023). A federal court blocks California's new medical misinformation law. *The New York Times*, January 26, 2023. https://www.nytimes.com/2023/01/26/technology/federal-court-blocks-california-medical-misinformation-law.html

National Academy of Medicine. (2017). *Communities in action: Pathways to equity.* National Academies Press. https://www.ncbi.nlm.nih.gov/books/NBK425851/

National Academy of Medicine. (2019). *Integrating social care into the delivery of health care: Moving upstream to improve the nation's health.* National Academies Press. https://www.nationalacademies.org/our-work/integrating-social-needs-care-into-the-delivery-of-health-care-to-improve-the-nations-health

National Academy of Medicine. (2020). *Evidence-based practice for public health emergency preparedness and response.* National Academies Press. https://www.nationalacademies.org/our-work/evidence-based-practices-for-public-health-emergency-preparedness-and-response-assessment-of-and-recommendations-for-the-field

National Academy of Medicine. (2021). *The future of nursing 2020–2030. Charting a path to achieve health equity.* https://nam.edu/publications/the-future-of-nursing-2020-2030/

National Institutes of Health. (2023a). *Policy.* U.S. Department of Health and Human Services. https://www.nih.gov/institutes-nih/nih-office-director/policy

National Institutes of Health. (2023b). *NIH-funded study highlights the financial toll of health disparities in the United States.* U.S. Department of Health and Human Services. https://www.nih.gov/news-events/news-releases/nih-funded-study-highlights-financial-toll-health-disparities-united-states

National Institute for Nursing Research. (2023). *News and events.* https://www.ninr.nih.gov/

National League for Nursing. (2023). *Public policy agenda.* https://www.nln.org/docs/default-source/default-document-library/2023-2024-nln-public-policy-agenda.pdf?sfvrsn=43753085_3

Nelson, R. (2021). Controversy over public health authority. *The American Journal of Nursing, 121*(11), 14.

Office of Disease Prevention and Health Promotion. (2015). *Health literacy online: A guide to simplifying the user experience.* U.S. Department of Health and Human Services. https://health.gov/healthliteracyonline/

Office of Disease Prevention and Health Promotion. (2020). *Health policy.* U.S. Department of Health and Human Services. https://health.gov/healthypeople/objectives-and-data/browse-objectives/health-policy

Office of Disease Prevention and Health Promotion. (2021). *About ODPHP.* U.S. Department of Health and Human Services. https://health.gov/about-odphp

Office of Minority Health. (2023). *The national CLAS standards.* U.S. Department of Health and Human Services. https://thinkculturalhealth.hhs.gov/clas/standards

Parmet, W. (2022). Fights between U.S. states and the national government are endangering public health. *Scientific American.* https://www.scientificamerican.com/article/fights-between-u-s-states-and-the-national-government-are-endangering-public-health/

Pew Research Center. (2023). *Social media fact sheet.* https://www.pewresearch.org/internet/factsheet/social-media/

Roberts, E. T., Kwon, Y., Hames, A. G., et al. (2023). Racial and ethnic disparities in health care use and access associated with loss of Medicaid supplemental insurance eligibility above the federal poverty level. *JAMA Internal Medicine, 183*(6), 534–543. https://jamanetwork.com/journals/jamainternalmedicine/article-abstract/2803780

Sisnowski, J., & Street, J. M. (2017). Evidence-informed public health policy. In S. R. Quah & W. C. Cockerham (Eds.), *International Encyclopedia of Public Health* (2nd ed.; pp. 527–536). https://doi.org/10.1016/B978-0-12-803678-5.00150-8

Summers, L., & Gordon, K. (2022). Is there a nurse in the House? Or the Senate? *American Nurse Journal*, October 5, 2022. https://www.myamericannurse.com/is-there-a-nurse-in-the-house-or-the-senate/?partnerref=Nurseline+20221011&utm_source=sfmc&utm_medium=email&utm_campaign=Nurseline+20221011&utm_term=https%3a%2f%2fwww.myamericannurse.com%2fis-there-a-nurse-in-the-house-or-the-senate%2f&utm id=17780&sfmc_id=11576504

Teitelbaum, J., McGowan, A. K., Richmond, T. S., et al. (2021). Law and policy as tools in Healthy People 2030. *Journal of Public Health Management Practice, 27*(6), S265–S273. https://doi.org/10.1097%2FPHH.0000000000001358

Twum-Danso, N. (2022). *Strengthening the connections between health care and public health*. Institute for Healthcare Improvement. https://www.ihi.org/communities/blogs/strengthening-the-connections-between-health-care-and-public-health?utm_campaign=tw&utm_medium=email&_hsmi=208860374&_hsenc=p2ANqtz-_el6Txqt-n37mfJ7SdFTrVfpblyn_I5t7-ANd5BXlVpmeOM8NlKRJ7GLA8HDq7AchK7I1SSi3R-ouJX3M2U8CW1k_LOI0g&utm_content=208737229&utm_source=hs_email

USAspending.gov. (2023). *U.S. Department of Health and Human Services (HHS)*. https://www.usaspending.gov/agency/department-of-health-and-human-services?fy=2023

U.S. Congress. (2023). *The legislative process*. https://www.congress.gov/legislative-process

U.S. Department of Health and Human Services. (2021). *Health literacy*. https://health.gov/our-work/national-health-initiatives/health-literacy

U.S. Department of Health and Human Services. (2022a). *HHS equity action plan*. https://www.hhs.gov/sites/default/files/hhs-equity-action-plan.pdf

U.S. Department of Health and Human Services. (2022b). *Strategic plan FY 2022–2026*. https://www.hhs.gov/about/strategic-plan/2022-2026/index.html

U.S. Department of Health and Human Services. (2023a). *About HHS*. https://www.hhs.gov/about/index.html

U.S. Department of Health and Human Services. (2023b). *Health and Human Services agencies and offices*. https://www.hhs.gov/about/agencies/hhs-agencies-and-offices/index.html

U.S. Department of Health and Human Services. (2023c). *Pandemic and All Hazards Preparedness Act*. https://aspr.hhs.gov/legal/pahpa/Pages/default.aspx

U.S. Department of Health and Human Services. (2023d). *HHS announces nearly $9 million to increase the number of substance use disorder clinicians in underserved communities*. https://www.hhs.gov/about/news/2023/06/14/hhs-announces-nearly-9-million-to-increase-the-number-of-substance-use-disorder-clinicians-in-underserved-communities.html?utm_campaign=enews20230615&utm_medium=email&utm_source=govdelivery

U.S. Department of Health and Human Services. (2023e). *HHS announces new $15 million loan repayment program to strengthen the pediatric health care workforce.* https://www.hhs.gov/about/news/2023/06/09/hhs-announces-new-15-million-loan-repayment-program-strengthen-pediatric-health-care-workforce.html?utm_campaign=enews20230615&utm_medium=email&utm_source=govdelivery

U.S. Department of Health and Human Services. (2023f). *Biden-Harris administration celebrates the Affordable Care Act's 13th anniversary and highlights record-breaking coverage.* https://www.hhs.gov/about/news/2023/03/23/biden-harris-administration-celebrates-affordable-care-acts-13th-anniversary-highlights-record-breaking-coverage.html

U.S. Department of Health and Human Services. (2023g). *Artificial intelligence (AI) at HHS.* https://www.hhs.gov/about/agencies/asa/ocio/ai/index.html

U.S. Department of Health and Human Services. (2023h). *Telehealth policy.* https://telehealth.hhs.gov/providers/policy-changes-during-the-covid-19-public-health-emergency

U.S. Department of the Treasury. (2020). *CARES Act of 2020.* https://home.treasury.gov/policy-issues/coronavirus/about-the-cares-act

U.S. Government Accountability Office. (2022). *COVID-19: Pandemic lessons highlight need for public health situational awareness network.* https://www.gao.gov/assets/gao-22-104600.pdf

U.S. Senate Committee on Homeland Security and Governmental Affairs. (2023). *Short supply: The health and national security risks of drug shortages.* https://www.hsgac.senate.gov/wp-content/uploads/2023-03-20-HSGAC-Majority-Draft-Drug-Shortages-Report.pdf

Valdez, R. (2023). *The end of the public health emergency refocuses the urgency to improve healthcare quality.* AHRQ Views, May 19, 2023. https://www.ahrq.gov/news/blog/ahrqviews/public-health-emergency-refocus.html

World Health Organization. (2023a). *Our work.* https://www.who.int/our-work

World Health Organization. (2023b). *WHO launches global network to detect and prevent infectious disease threats.* https://www.who.int/news/item/20-05-2023-who-launches-global-network-to--detect-and-prevent-infectious-disease-threats

Wyatt, R., Laderman, M., Botwinick, L., Mate, K., & Whittington. J. (2016). *Achieving health equity: A guide for health care organizations.* Institute for Healthcare Improvement white paper. http://www.ihi.org/resources/Pages/IHIWhitePapers/Achieving-Health-Equity.aspx

Figure Credits

Fig. 1: Source: https://www.cdc.gov/surveillance/pdfs/318212-A_DMI_LogicModel_July23b-508.pdf?utm_source=substack&utm_medium=email.

Fig. 2: Source: https://www.gao.gov/products/gao-22-104600.

Fig. 3: Source: https://www.cdc.gov/about/sdoh/index.html.

Fig. 4: Source: https://www.cdc.gov/policy/hi5/index.html.

Fig. 5: Source: https://www.cdc.gov/policy/polaris/policyprocess/strategy-development/index.html.

Fig. 6: Source: https://www.congress.gov/legislative-process.

Fig. 7: Source: https://www.cdc.gov/policy/polaris/training/writing-briefs/index.html.

Fig. 8: Source: https://www.cdc.gov/policy/hiap/index.html.

Fig. 9: The Office of the National Coordinator for Health Information Technology, https://www.healthit.gov/sites/default/files/page/2020-10/Federal%20Health%20IT%20Strategic%20Plan_2020_2025.pdf, 2020, p. 4.

Fig. 10: U.S. Department of Health and Human Services, A Guide for Rural Health Care Collaboration and Coordination, https://www.hrsa.gov/sites/default/files/hrsa/rural-health/resources/hrsa-rural-collaboration-guide.pdf, 2019, p. 4.

Appendix A

Public and Community Health: Framework and Concepts

The following content provides some basic information and terminology related to public and community health.

Public and Community Health

Public health is the area of health care that focuses on prevention and control of disease and disability, with particular concern for groups (i.e., populations and communities). Healthy behaviors and wellness are important for public health. **Figure A.1** identifies the major core sciences that are associated with public health and used to meet its goals.

Community health focuses on providing comprehensive accessible services to a community to ensure health needs are met, considers social determinants of health that affect the community, and aims to reduce health disparities while supporting health equity. The latter aim involves an increased emphasis on advocacy and policy development and implementation to ensure a healthy community.

Who Does Public and Community Health Serve?

Within public and community health, various terms are used to identify those who need assistance. Examples of these terms include:

- *Individuals* (also *patients, clients*, and *consumers*)
- *Families*
- *Aggregates* or *populations*
- *Communities*

The public and community health focus is less on individuals and more on groups (e.g., families; populations, such as persons with heart disease; and communities).

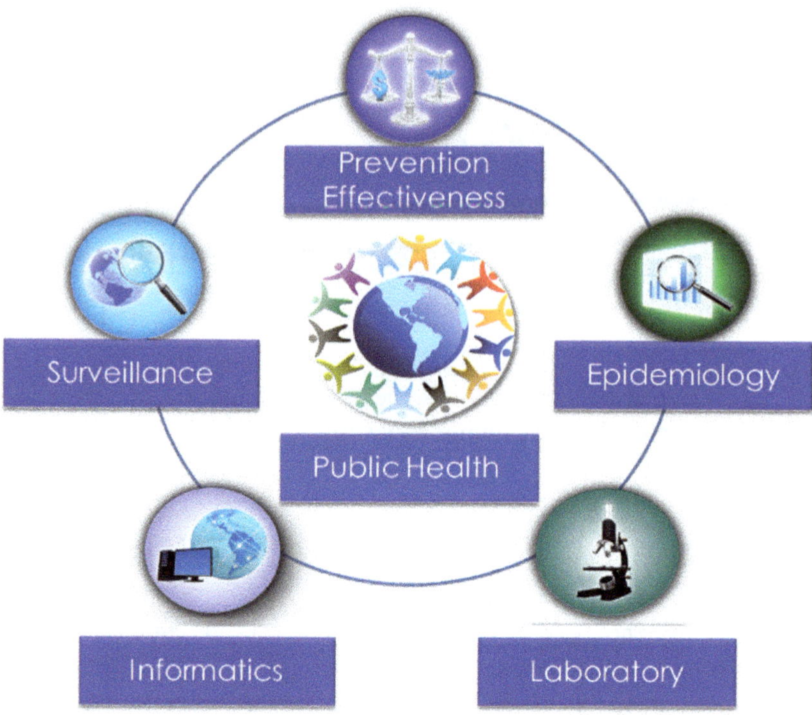

Figure A.1. Public Health Core Sciences

Healthcare Providers

Healthcare providers are individuals and organizations providing health services. Examples of individuals are professionals such as physicians, registered nurses, pharmacists, social workers, and others (e.g., nutritionists, government health inspectors [food, business safety], health educators, community planners, epidemiologists, public policymakers, school health staff, community first responders). Healthcare organizations include acute care hospitals, clinics, community-based service agencies, home healthcare agencies, centers providing urgent care and emergency services, and pharmacies. In communities, health departments and their associated services, such as clinics and often school health, provide critical services to the community. Within business and industry, occupational health services offer support for employees and health education and prevention and have an impact on the overall health of the community.

Groups and Teams

In this guide, the term *team* is used rather than *group*. Within healthcare (e.g., acute care, community health, and public health), *team* is more commonly used; staff are members of teams in their workplaces. Students need to become familiar with this term, and to encourage this perspective, the guide refers to student *teams* rather than *groups*.

The Public Health Model

There are three public health core functions:

- **Assessment:** Relates to essential services 1–2
- **Policy development:** Relates to essential services 3–5
- **Assurance:** Relates to essential services 6–10

Nurses who work in public and community health are involved in each of the three core functions and the following 10 public health essential services:

1. Assess and monitor population health status, factors that influence health, and community needs and assets.
2. Investigate, diagnose, and address health problems and hazards affecting the population.
3. Communicate effectively to inform and educate people about health, factors that influence it, and how to improve it.
4. Strengthen, support, and mobilize communities and partnerships to improve health.
5. Create, champion, and implement policies, plans, and laws that impact health.
6. Utilize legal and regulatory actions designed to improve and protect the public's health.
7. Ensure an effective system that enables equitable access to the individual services and care needed to be healthy.
8. Build and support a diverse and skilled public health workforce
9. Improve and innovate public health functions through ongoing evaluation, research, and continuous quality improvement.
10. Build and maintain a strong organizational infrastructure for public health.

Figure A.2 describes the interrelationship between the core functions and essential services.

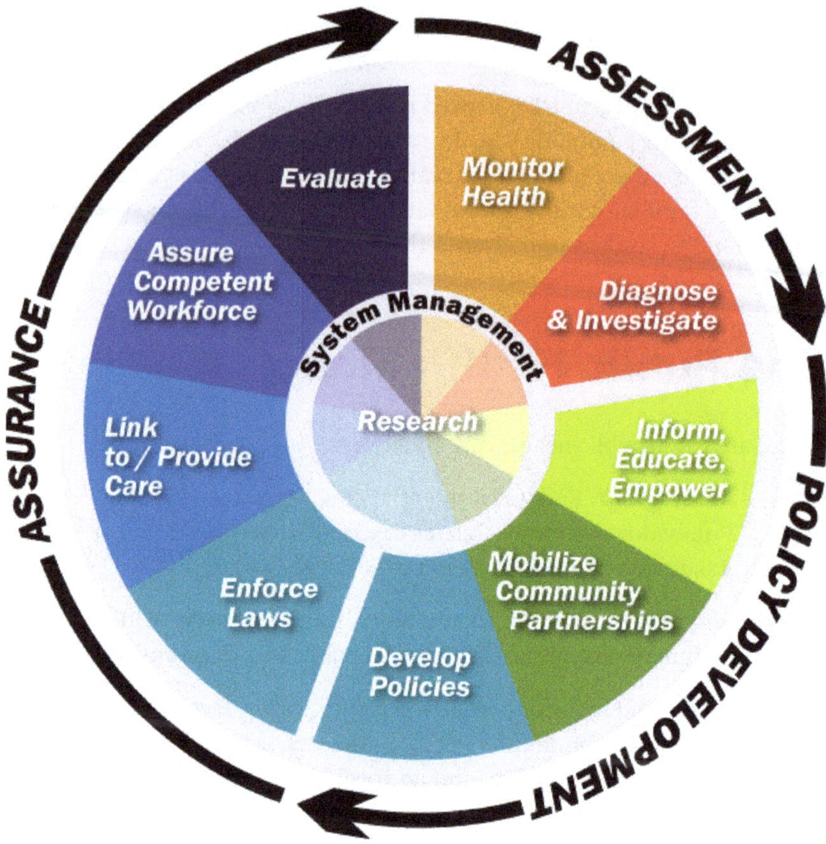

Figure A.2. Public Health Core Functions and Essential Services

Public Health Core Competencies

A collaborative of 24 national organizations concerned with public health education developed the following competencies. These are based on the 10 essential public health services and should be applied to all public health professionals. The goal of this collaboration is to improve public health by ensuring competent staff and effective healthcare organization performance. Identification of these competencies also recognizes the need for effective coordination and monitoring of outcomes among the key stakeholders in academic institutions, public health practice, and healthcare communities. Education must include not only preparation education but also ongoing staff education at the work site. The collaboration also notes that there is an ongoing need to develop effective strategies for positive public health outcomes. The following describes the domains—specific activity areas—emphasized in these core competencies:

Domain 1: Data Analytics and Assessment Skills

Focuses on factors that affect the health of the community, data collection, analysis of data, use of public health informatics applying data and information, assessment of community health status

Domain 2: Policy Development and Program Planning Skills

Development, implementation, and evaluation of policies, programs, and services to improve

Domain 3: Communication Skills

Strategies for internal and external use; responding to information, including misinformation and disinformation; facilitating individual, group, and organization communication

Domain 4: Health Equity Skills

Effective use of principles related to ethics, diversity, equity, inclusion, and justice; self-awareness of biases; working effectively in diverse situations and with diverse people to reduce systematic and structural barriers while advocating for health equity

Domain 5: Community Partnership Skills

Establishing community relationships and working to improve community health and resilience; collaborating and sharing power

Domain 6: Public Health Science Skills

With an understanding of systems, policies, and situations that impact public health, applying the 10 essential public health services, evidence-based practice, and support research to provide more evidence for public health practice

Domain 7: Management and Finance Skills

Effectively applying basic management and finance skills to public health, such as planning, quality, human resources, staff development, finance, policies, integration of diversity, teams and teamwork, collaboration, performance management, using the healthy community model, and application of three public health core functions and 10 essential services

Domain 8: Leadership and Systems-Thinking Skills

Identifies facilitators and barriers related to 10 essential public health services; serves as leader to encourage creativity, innovation, responding to current trends, directing effective change, collaborating with stakeholders in the community, and advocating for public health

Nurses must also follow relevant nursing standards and competencies.

Source: Council on Linkages Between Academia and Public Health Practice. (2021, October). *Core competencies for public health professionals.* http://www.phf.org/resourcestools/pages/core_public_health_competencies.aspx

The nursing profession responded to the development of the above public heath core competencies by aligning public health nursing competencies with them. The nursing competencies focus on public health nursing practice, from entry level to senior nursing management positions, and integrate the competencies that were developed for all public health professionals. There are also eight domains in the public health nursing competencies. Given that the focus in this guide is on health equity and disparities, domains that are particularly related to these issues are identified as follows, although many of the other domains are indirectly related to this content (Quad Council Coalition, 2018):

- **Cultural competency skills** focus on understanding and responding to diverse needs, assessing organizational cultural diversity and competence, assessing effects of policies and programs on various populations, and taking action to support a diverse public health workforce (relates to Domain 4).
- **Community dimensions of practice skills** focus on evaluating and developing linkages and relationships within the community, maintaining and advancing partnerships and community involvement, negotiating for the use of community assets, defending public health policies and programs, and evaluating and improving the effectiveness of community engagement (relates to Domain 5).

Source: Quad Council Coalition. (2018). *Community/public health nursing [C/PHN] competencies.* https://www.cphno.org/wp-content/uploads/2020/08/QCC-C-PHN-COMPETENCIES-Approved_2018.05.04_Final-002.pdf

Public Health Nursing Standards

The American Nurses Association (ANA) has developed and updated standards for many specialties. *Public Health Nursing: Scope & Standards of Practice* includes standards related to the following: assessment, population diagnosis and priorities, outcomes identification, planning, implementation, coordination of care, health teaching and health promotion, consultation, prescriptive authority, regulatory activities, evaluation, professional performance for public health nursing, ethics, evidence-based practice and research, quality of practice, communication, leadership, collaboration, professional practice evaluation, resource utilization, environmental health, and advocacy. As is true for all ANA standards and as is mentioned in the guide's content, health equity is an important concern.

Source: *American Nurses Association.* (2022). Public health nursing: Scope & standards of practice (3rd ed.). https://www.nursingworld.org/nurses-books/public-health-nursing–scope–standards-of-practice-2nd-edition/

An example of other standards that relate to public and community health are the American Academy of Ambulatory Care Nursing (AAACN) *Scope and Standards of Telehealth Nursing.* The AAACN recognizes that telehealth/digital health is important in ambulatory care. The AAACN standards defines telehealth, in acute care and public and community health, as "nursing practice using the nursing process to provide care for individual patients or defined patient populations through telecommunications media" (American Academy of Ambulatory Care Nursing, 2018, p. 10).

References

American Academy of Ambulatory Care Nursing. (2018). *Scope and standards of practice for professional telehealth nursing* (6th ed.). https://www.aaacn.org/practice-resources/telehealth/scope-and-standards

American Nurses Association. (2022). *Public health nursing: Scope and standards of practice* (3rd ed.). https://www.nursingworld.org/nurses-books/public-health-nursing-scope-and-standards-of-prac/

Council on Linkages Between Academia and Public Health Practice. (2021, October). *Core competencies for public health professionals*. http://www.phf.org/resourcestools/pages/core_public_health_competencies.aspx

Quad Council Coalition. (2018). *Community/public health nursing [C/PHN] competencies*. https://www.cphno.org/wp-content/uploads/2020/08/QCC-C-PHN-COMPETENCIES-Approved_2018.05.04_Final-002.pdf

Figure Credits

Fig. A.1: Source: https://www.cdc.gov/training/publichealth101/documents/introduction-to-public-health.pdf.

Fig. A.2: Source: https://www.cdc.gov/publichealthgateway/publichealthservices/originalessentialhealthservices.html.

Appendix B

The National Initiative to Improve the Nation's Health: Healthy People 2030

The U.S. Department of Health and Human Services (HHS), its agencies, and other government departments are responsible for assessing and developing plans and resources to ensure the health of all people who live in the United States by promoting health and preventing disease and illness. HHS works with healthcare services at the federal, state, and local levels. As part of this responsibility, Healthy People 2030 is a major federal program that provides a comprehensive plan focused on health promotion and disease prevention and routinely assesses national health status. The initiative is reviewed and updated every 10 years, with five past editions (1979, 1990, 2000, 2010, and 2020) and the current edition, which is due to end in 2030. The latest version's vision and major goals focus on the topics of health conditions, health behaviors, populations, settings and systems, and social determinants of health (SDOH).

Health status is determined by measuring birth and death rates, life expectancy, quality of life, morbidity from specific diseases, risk factors, use of ambulatory care and inpatient care, accessibility to health providers and facilities, financing of healthcare services, health insurance coverage, access to healthcare, and other factors. Quality is a complex healthcare issue that affects the health status of individuals and communities. There is not one single factor or behavior that determines outcomes, but rather multiple factors—such as genetics, lifestyle, gender, race/ethnic factors, nutrition, poverty level, education, environment, injury, violence, environment, and unavailability or inaccessibility of high-quality health services.

Healthy People 2030 Framework

Vision

A society in which all people can achieve their full potential for health and well-being across the lifespan.

Mission

To promote, strengthen, and evaluate the nation's efforts to improve the health and well-being of all people.

Foundational Principles

Foundational principles explain the thinking that guides decisions about Healthy People 2030:

- Health and well-being of all people and communities are essential to a thriving, equitable society.
- Promoting health and well-being and preventing disease are linked efforts that encompass physical, mental, and social health dimensions.
- Investing to achieve the full potential for health and well-being for all provides valuable benefits to society.
- Achieving health and well-being requires eliminating health disparities, achieving health equity, and attaining health literacy.
- Healthy physical, social, and economic environments strengthen the potential to achieve health and well-being.
- Promoting and achieving the nation's health and well-being is a shared responsibility that is distributed across the national, state, tribal, and community levels, including the public, private, and not-for-profit sectors.
- Working to attain the full potential for health and well-being of the population is a component of decision-making and policy formulation across all sectors.

Overarching Goals

- Attain healthy, thriving lives and well-being, free of preventable disease, disability, injury, and premature death.
- Eliminate health disparities, achieve health equity, and attain health literacy to improve the health and well-being of all.

Office of Disease Prevention and Health Promotion (ODPHP), Selections from "Healthy People 2030 Framework," https://health.gov/healthypeople/about/healthy-people-2030-framework, 2021.

- Create social, physical, and economic environments that promote attaining full potential for health and well-being for all.
- Promote healthy development and healthy behaviors and well-being across all life stages.
- Engage leadership, key constituents, and the public across multiple sectors to take action and design policies that improve the health and well-being of all.

Plan of Action

To achieve the health and well-being of all people, relevant stakeholders need to be active partners, across the public, private, and nonprofit sectors. Healthy People conducts regular monitoring of the plan's progress. The results are made public on its website.

The Healthy People objectives are developed to meet the overall goals and are based on data and changed as needed during each 10-year cycle. This includes eight broad outcome measures used to assess the program's vision, 355 measurable core public health objectives with 10-year targets and related evidence-based interventions, developmental goals for public health issues with interventions, and research objectives directed at public health issues for which there are no evidence-based interventions.

Healthy People 2030 focuses on individual health and on communities. It describes a healthy community as one that maintains a high quality of life and is productive and safe, provides both treatment and prevention services to all community members, maintains necessary effective infrastructure (e.g., water, energy, roads, transportation, schools, playgrounds, and other services), and maintains a healthy environment (for example, issues of pollution, such as with air and water). Educational and community-based programs need to focus on preventing disease and injury, promoting and improving health, and enhancing quality of life. This view of a healthy community relates to the SDOH.

To meet Healthy People goals, community programs and services must provide broad access (e.g., located in schools, workplaces, healthcare facilities, and community sites) and offer prevention, monitoring, treatment, and rehabilitation services.

The Healthy People 2030 initiative not only provides a 10-year plan to improve healthcare in the United States but also monitors and reports on progress by assessing the outcome status of its goals and objectives. Data on current outcomes can be found on the Healthy People website. At the end of the 10-year period, all outcomes are evaluated and summarized. This information is then used to develop the plan for the next 10 years—the goals, objectives, and leading indicators.

Stakeholders

Many organizations, government, and individuals are involved in the development, implementation, and evaluation of the Healthy People initiative. Nurses need to understand the importance of stakeholders so that they can collaborate with relevant stakeholders and advocate for healthy communities. **Figure B.1** describes the Healthy People stakeholders.

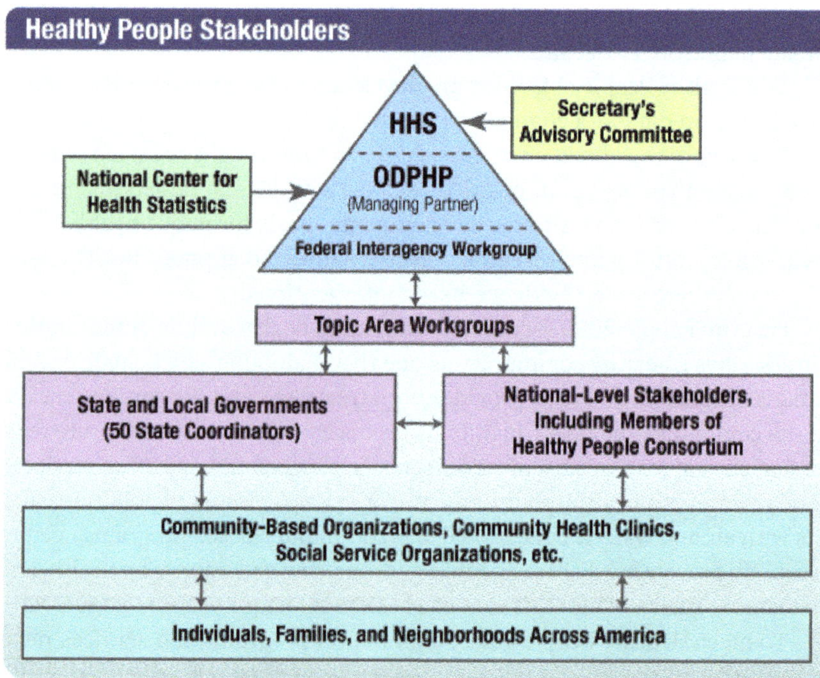

Figure B.1. Healthy People Stakeholders

Healthy People 2030: Emergency Preparedness

See information about emergency preparedness and updates on this topic at https://health.gov/healthypeople/objectives-and-data/browse-objectives/emergency-preparedness.

Healthy People 2030: Current Information

- Explore the leading health Indicators used by Healthy People to monitor its outcomes.
  Source: https://health.gov/healthypeople/objectives-and-data
- Explore SDOH and relationship to Healthy People.
  Source: https://health.gov/healthypeople/objectives-and-data
- Explore overall health and well-being measures.
  Source: https://health.gov/healthypeople/objectives-and-data
- Explore new objectives.
  Source: https://health.gov/news/202207/check-out-healthy-people-2030s-new-objectives?source=govdelivery&utm_medium=email&utm_source=govdelivery

References

U.S. Department of Health and Human Services, Office of Disease Prevention and Health Promotion. (2023). *Healthy People 2030*. https://health.gov/healthypeople

U.S. Department of Health and Human Services, Office of Disease Prevention and Health Promotion. (2023). *Tools for action*. Healthy People 2030. https://health.gov/healthypeople/tools-action

Figure Credit

Fig. B.1: Source: https://www.cdc.gov/nchs/about/factsheets/factsheet-hp2030.htm.

Appendix C

Institute of Medicine/National Academy of Medicine Reports

The National Academy of Medicine (NAM) is the former Institute of Medicine (IOM), and since 2015, it has been referred to as the *NAM*. The IOM/NAM has provided significant examination of healthcare issues and expert advice to healthcare organizations, individual providers, and health policymakers, both governmental and nongovernmental (NAM, 2021). The IOM/NAM is a nongovernmental, nonprofit organization that was created in 1970. Why is it mentioned in this guide, which deals with equity and disparities? Its reports cover many topics, some of which are relevant to this content. The NAM asks experts to examine an issue, provides staff and funding for the review, and then publishes information from the review and often identifies recommendations (Finkelman, 2017). These recommendations are not laws or regulations, but they often have a major impact on healthcare decision-making.

The following are brief summaries of early reports that had a significant influence on how the nation's healthcare delivery system and health policy view quality care as well as more current reports that highlight some areas of interest to this guide's content. Some of the reports are mentioned within the guide's content.

To Err Is Human **(1999)** Due to growing questions about quality care, President William Clinton's Advisory Commission on Consumer Protection and Quality in the Health Care Industry stimulated further examination of quality and asked the IOM to further examine healthcare, focusing on errors. The report from this request, *To Err Is Human*, stirred a strong reaction by indicating that there were many errors in the U.S. healthcare system. The results were widely discussed in the media, so consumers became more aware of this problem. In addition, the report emphasized that the healthcare delivery system put too much emphasis on blame for errors, particularly on individual staff. This led to an active initiative to alter this approach.

Most errors are system errors, not individuals making mistakes. The report focused on acute care.

Crossing the Quality Chasm **(2001)** A second major report on healthcare quality followed *To Err Is Human*. It focused on broader issues of quality care and concluded that more information was needed. This report also focused on acute care. Even with President Bill Clinton's commission's review and two extensive reviews and reports on healthcare quality, there was still concern that we did not know enough, and the problem was extensive. Public and community health also needed to be examined, and later reports included this vital health care area.

Envisioning the National Healthcare Quality Report **(2001)** The 1999 and 2001 reports mentioned earlier identified the need for systematic monitoring of healthcare quality to better understand the status of quality care. This monitoring needed to be done routinely and include analysis and recommendations for improvement. *Envisioning the National Healthcare Quality Report* described an initial framework for the new annual monitoring process and report. The Agency for Healthcare Research and Quality, an agency within the U.S. Department of Health and Human Services (HHS), is responsible for this annual report (titled the *National Healthcare Quality and Disparities Report* [NHQDR]), which initially focused solely on quality care.

Unequal Treatment: Confronting Racial and Ethnic Disparities in Health Care **(2003)** This report began to expand the healthcare perspective by including more about public and community health. As more was learned about quality care, it became clear that there were health disparities due in particular to bias, prejudice, and stereotyping. Just as with the issue of quality care, there was a need to monitor disparities, and this led to the development of a monitoring system and report similar to the NHQDR, which was later combined with the quality report.

Health Professions Education: A Bridge to Quality **(2003)** This report moved the quality care discussion to health professions education. With the growing recognition that care needed to improve, which required routine monitoring and improvement, it was determined that a key ingredient to accomplishing this objective were the staff—namely, whether they were prepared to provide effective and efficient care to diverse populations. This conclusion and the report were critical in that the recommendations included five core competencies that all healthcare professionals should meet. It is significant that the experts decided to identify competencies that did not focus on one healthcare profession. These competencies are as follows:

1. Provide patient-centered care (person-centered).
2. Work in interprofessional teams.
3. Employ evidence-based practice.
4. Apply quality improvement.
5. Utilize informatics.

Later, the nursing profession developed core competencies for nursing (Quality and Safety Education for nurses [QSEN]) that related to these core health profession competencies; however, it is important that nursing avoids separating itself from these core competencies. The major difference is that QSEN has six competencies and separates quality from safety, and the IOM/NAM recommendation on core competencies considers safety an integral part of quality.

Source: QSEN Institute (2020). *QSEN Institute competencies.* https://qsen.org/competencies/

Health Literacy **(2004)** With the goal of examining diversity and disparities, this report recognized that health literacy has a major impact on quality care and the health of individuals and communities.

Health Literacy: A Prescription to End Confusion **(2004)** Communication is critical in health care—both written and oral and with all stakeholders. This includes individuals, families, staff, communities, other professionals, and government, among others. Effective partnerships require effective, ongoing communication. When problems with communication occur, health literacy issues may arise. Understanding is necessary for effective healthcare decision-making—affecting locations to obtain treatment, treatment providers, types of treatment, the ability to follow treatment, the ability to engage in self-care, questions to ask healthcare providers, and so on. Yet, millions of Americans cannot understand or act upon this information. This report discussed health literacy and methods to improve communication for individuals and populations.

Keeping Patients Safe: Transforming the Work Environment for Nurses **(2004);** ***The Future of Nursing: Leading Change, Advancing Health*** **(2010);** ***The Future of Nursing 2020–2030: Charting a Path to Achieve Health Equity*** **(2020)** Some of the IOM/NAM reports have focused on nursing. One of the significant early reports was *Keeping Patients Safe: Transforming the Work Environment for Nurses*, which primarily discussed acute care nursing practice, particularly staff nurses and related workforce issues. In 2010, a landmark report titled *The Future of Nursing: Leading Change, Advancing Health* examined current and future roles of nurses. The third report mentioned Is directly related to the content of this guide, *The Future of Nursing 2020–2030: Charting a Path to Achieve Health Equity* (2020). These reports are discussed in relevant content in the guide.

***The Future of the Public's Health in the 21st Century* (2003) and *Who Will Keep the Public Healthy?* (2003)** The initial reports from the IOM focused on acute care, although some of the content could be applied to public and community health. There was slow recognition that separating acute care from public and community health or ignoring the healthcare delivery system as a whole was not effective. In 2003, this view changed with the publication of two key public and community health reports. *The Future of the Public's Health in the 21st Century* examined the need to apply a population health approach, develop effective public health infrastructure, establish partnerships, ensure accountability, implement evidence-based practice, and utilize clear communication. *Who Will Keep the Public Healthy?* turned the focus to identifying the public health competencies, which are related to informatics, genomics, communication, culture, community-based participatory research, global health, policy and law, and public health ethics. The report provided a guide for public and community health education content, such as for nursing.

***Informed Consent and Health Literacy* (2015)** This report discussed a specific issue related to health literacy, which by 2015 had been recognized as a major concern in healthcare delivery. Participants in research are asked to sign a consent form, and agreeing to do so should be an informed decision. In order to be able to make this decision, participants must understand the information they are given. Ensuring that participants can agree and understand prior to participating in a research study is a critical part of ethics and participant rights.

***Health Literacy: Past, Present, and Future* (2015)** Given the concern about health literacy, this report examined the problems, origins, and consequences of adult health literacy. Adults who do not have the required level of health literacy may not be able to engage safely in their own health and healthcare decision-making. The report includes solutions such as the need for organizational changes, including system changes to assist in reducing health literacy.

***A Framework for Educating Health Professionals to Address Social Determinants of Health* (2016)** As more has been learned about the importance of the social determinants of health (SDOH), there has been growing recognition that healthcare professionals need to learn about these determinants so that they are more aware of the impact on health and disparities. From this, healthcare professionals will then be better able to intervene and improve the health of individuals, communities, and populations.

Collaboration Between Health Care and Public Health (2016) This report discussed the need for effective collaboration between acute health care and public health. This partnership needs to include shared goals, community engagement, aligned leadership, sustainability, and data and analysis. There are barriers to this collaboration, including inadequate communication, working with interprofessional teams, and understanding diverse cultures, among others, that must be addressed.

Communities in Action: Pathways to Health Equity (2017) This report continued to examine health equity, disparities, and the SDOH. It particularly noted that we know individual behavior and health status are important, but there is also a need to view these issues from a community perspective. It is the community that has a strong impact on poverty, unemployment, poor education, inadequate housing, poor public transportation, interpersonal violence, and struggling neighborhoods, all of which influence health. Social policies also make a difference in inequalities and contribute to health inequities. The report examined the causes of and possible solutions to health inequities, emphasizing the importance of communities in promoting health equity.

Perspectives on Health Equity and Social Determinants of Health (2017) This report examined the social factors that influence the nation's health (i.e., the SDOH); racism and poverty, which result in inequitable social, environmental, and economic conditions; and health disparities. It included content on policies and strategies used to address these problems, focusing on the need for collective actions.

Community-Based Health Literacy Interventions (2018) This report focused on community interventions to reduce health literacy problems, examining types of community-based literacy interventions and methods to evaluate their results and providing examples. Community infrastructure and staff are critical elements to success, as is a commitment to improve community trust.

Immigration as a Social Determinant of Health (2018) The United States has a large immigrant population, which experiences systematic marginalization and discrimination that often result in health disparities. This report examined the relationship between the immigration experience and health outcomes.

Improving Access to and Equity of Care for People With Serious Illness: Proceedings of a Workshop **(2019)** At the time this report was completed, the Centers for Disease Control and Prevention (CDC) estimated that approximately 40 million people in the United States had a serious illness. This type of disease limits daily activities. As health disparities were examined, it was noted that this population also experiences disparities due to race, ethnicity, gender, geography, and socioeconomic and insurance status. This is found in multiple communities and interferes with healthcare access and quality. Improvement requires engagement and feedback from individuals (patient and family), healthcare providers, organizations, and communities.

Integrating Social Care Into the Delivery of Health Care: Moving Upstream to Improve the Nation's Health **(2019)** With the recognition of the importance of the SDOH in regards to health equity and disparities, the healthcare delivery system must turn to improvement. The key questions addressed in this report were as follows:

- How can services that address social needs be integrated into clinical care?
- What type of infrastructure will be needed to facilitate that integration?

The report concluded that five complementary activities should be used ensure integration of social care into health care: awareness, adjustment, assistance, alignment, and advocacy. The report discussed these activities and stated that they should be used by healthcare organizations and providers, communities, social services, and governments.

Population Health in Rural America **(2020)** Rural areas of the United States experience many health problems and difficulties with receiving effective and timely health care. People who live in rural areas are a vulnerable and diverse population. Rural areas also experience serious healthcare delivery problems, such as a shortage of healthcare professionals and services.

Population Health in Challenging Times: Insights From Key Domains: Proceedings of a Workshop **(2021)** This report examined population health, which is a complex area of health care. The workshop identified key areas of concern in population health and underscored the fact that this type of health is a significant issue in the nation's health.

Priorities on the Health Horizon: Informing PCORI's Strategic Plan (2021) This report discussed the need for more evidence to support healthcare delivery and practice. It particularly focused on equitable, stakeholder-driven, evidence-guided, patient-centered care. All of this requires effective collaborative relationships between patients, families, clinicians, healthcare administrators, researchers, and policymakers. PCORI is the Patient-Centered Outcomes Research Institute, an independent nonprofit, nongovernmental organization in Washington, D.C., that was authorized by Congress in 2010 to address the gap in information needed to make effective healthcare decisions. For more information, visit https://www.pcori.org/about/about-pcori.

Dialogue About the Workforce for Population Health Improvement: Proceedings of a Workshop (2021) This workshop focused on the needs of the population health workforce to improve health. Some of the discussion topics included peer-to-peer chronic disease management educators, health navigators, community health workers, public and health and healthcare leaders, developing competencies of the nonmedical and nonpublic health workforce, and application of the Health in All Policies model.

Exploring the Role of Critical Health Literacy in Addressing the Social Determinants of Health: Proceedings of a Workshop in Brief (2021) Due to growing concern about the SDOH, a discussion and subsequent report focused on this issue. It particularly addressed the impact of health literacy on the SDOH and vulnerable populations. The emphasis was on using literacy strategies to support effective health literacy associated with the SDOH.

To Achieve Health Equity, Leverage Nurses and Increase Funding for School and Public Health Nursing (2022) This report focused on nursing, but rather than discussing acute care, it examined the roles of nursing in public health, driven by the need to improve health equity. Improvements in public health nursing education are needed. The key recommendations are for the next 10 years included:

- Strengthening nursing education
- Promoting diversity, inclusivity, and equity in nursing education and the workforce
- Investing in school and public health nurses
- Protecting nurses' health and well-being

- Preparing nurses for disaster and public health emergency response
- Increasing the number of PhD-prepared nurses

Reducing Inequalities Between Lesbian, Gay, Bisexual, Transgender, and Queer Adolescents and Cisgender, Heterosexual Adolescents: Proceedings of a Workshop (2022) Lesbian, gay, bisexual, transgender, and queer as well as cisgender, heterosexual adolescents are at risk for health and social problems. As a vulnerable population, they require assessment and interventions that address health equity and reduce disparities. This report examined these concerns.

Realizing the Promise of Equity in the Organ Transplantation System (2022) Organ transplantation is a complex healthcare need that is supported by a complex system. A key concern is health equities and disparities for some who need this care. This report discussed the many issues patients and families experience and the system that supports organ transplantation.

Closing Evidence Gaps in Clinical Prevention (2022) This report examined the need for more research to provide evidence supporting effective clinical prevention working in collaboration with the HHS and the U.S. Preventive Services Task Force. For more information, visit https://www.ahrq.gov/cpi/about/otherwebsites/uspstf/index.html.

Measuring Sex, Gender Identity, and Sexual Orientation (2022) This report explored current information on the topics of sex, gender identity, and sexual orientation, highlighting the importance of tackling issues related to this population.

Healthy, Resilient, and Sustainable Communities After Disasters (2015) Communities must recover after disasters and work with multiple stakeholders to rebuild and repair infrastructure, provide health and social services, and supply new resources. Equitable access is a critical element.

Community Power in Population Health Improvement (2022) Community power is required to assess and improve population health within a community. This report discussed various actions that might be taken, including with education, transportation, environmental health, healthy eating, and active living.

Rapid Expert Consultation on Crisis Standards of Care for the COVID-19 Pandemic (2021) Crisis standards of care are not new, but during the

COVID-19 pandemic, more consumers and healthcare providers and organizations became familiar with them and their implications. They were applied in many states and had an impact on who received care and when. These issues are examined in this report.

Lessons Learned in Health Professions Education During the COVID-19 Pandemic, Parts 1 and 2 (2021; 2022) This report examines the issues and challenges that healthcare professions education confronted during COVID-19. Experts discussed the experience and made recommendations that should apply across varied healthcare professions.

Implementing High-Quality Primary Care: Rebuilding the Foundation of Health Care (2021) High-quality primary care is important for an effective healthcare system. It should provide continuous, person-centered, relationship-based care that considers the needs and preferences of individuals, families, and communities. Primary care is necessary to prevent health problems from becoming more serious and reducing need for more extensive healthcare services and reducing costs.

Integrating the Patient and Caregiver Voice in Serious Illness (2017) This report discusses the need for overall care quality through the delivery of person-centered and family-oriented services, for patients of all ages and across disease stages, care settings, and specialties. The increasing number of older adults represent a vulnerable population that requires health system support, and other services to meet their complex needs can be found across the age spectrum and in a broad range of care settings, from perinatal care to geriatric care.

Caring for People With Serious Illness: Lessons Learned From the COVID-19 Pandemic: Proceedings of a Workshop (2022) This report discussed the impact of the COVID-19 pandemic, noting ongoing weaknesses in the U.S. healthcare system and the need to address challenges related to caring for people with serious illness. Some of these issues include the use of healthcare teams providing care to people with serious illness, the impact of the pandemic on the healthcare workforce, the use of telehealth, issues related to clearly communication with the public about health emergencies, policy opportunities to improve care for people with serious illness, and health equity.

Models for Population Health Improvement by Health Care Systems and Partners: Tensions and Promise on the Path Upstream (2022) The CDC instituted a reevaluation of many of its activities for current disease control mechanisms, including the use of quarantine as a public health tool. This report was part of this reevaluation. The CDC's assessment should consider disease management responsibilities and the federal quarantine station network in mitigating the risk of onward communicable disease transmission considering changes in the global environment, including large increases in international travel, threats posed by emerging infections, and the movement of animals and cargo.

"Reimagining Patient-Centered Care During a Pandemic in a Digital World: A Focus on Building Trust for Healing" (2021) This was not a full report but rather a commentary from the NAM on a critical topic: patient-centered care during the COVID-19 pandemic and its relationship to digital health.

Source: Gupta, A., Cuff, P., Dotson-Blake, K., Schwartzberg, J., Sheperis, C., & Talib, Z. (2021). Reimagining patient-centered care during a pandemic in a digital world: A focus on building trust for healing. *NAM Perspectives.* Commentary, National Academy of Medicine, Washington, D.C. https://doi.org/10.31478/202105c

Global Roadmap for Healthy Longevity **(2022)** This report detailed planning to improve healthy longevity globally by 2050. It focused on a health approach with full inclusion of people of all ages, regardless of their health or functional status, in all aspects of society (e.g., education, work environment, health systems, aging and retirement, infrastructure, and physical environment), and societies characterized by social cohesion and equity—noting that health is interconnected with many factors.

Toward a Post-Pandemic World: Lessons From COVID-19 for Now and the Future: Proceedings of a Workshop **(2022)** This report discussed a workshop that focused on lessons learned from COVID-19 that should be considered by communities and healthcare providers to prepare for future public health crises. Data from this experience were applied to an examination of what happened as well as responses and outcomes.

Identifying Credible Sources of Health Information in Social Media: Principles and Attributes **(2022)** This paper discussed issues related to using social media in health areas, emphasizing the need for these sources to provide credible health information.

Source: Kington, R. S., Arnesen, S., Chou, W.-Y. S., Curry, S. J., Lazer, D., & Villarruel, A. M. (2021). Identifying credible sources of health information in social media: Principles and attributes. *NAM Perspectives.* Discussion paper, National Academy of Medicine, Washington, D.C. https://doi.org/10.31478/202107a

Innovations for Tackling Tuberculosis in the Time of COVID (2022) This report examined the global status of tuberculosis. During the COVID-19 pandemic, the rate of drug-resistant tuberculosis (TB) increased. TB is one of the deadliest communicable diseases in the world and has a major impact on poor communities and vulnerable populations. TB is also an example of how focus on a major pandemic can also negatively affect other global health problems.

The National Imperative to Improve Nursing Home Quality: Honoring Our Commitment to Residents, Families, and Staff (2022) Nursing homes are not just places where people receive care; these people also consider them their home. Quality is critical and crosses all aspects of the resident's life, not just health care. COVID-19 had an impact on nursing homes—specifically, how they function in public health emergencies, provide overall care, and meet daily needs. This is a challenge, and more needs to be learned from it so that this type of care can be improved.

Emerging Stronger From COVID-19: Priorities for Health System Transformation (2022) This report examined the COVID-19 public health emergency, its impact on the healthcare system, and the need for preparation and improvement.

Accelerating the Use of Findings From Patient-Centered Outcomes Research in Clinical Practice to Improve Health and Health Care: Proceedings of a Workshop Series (2022) This report examined the need for patient-centered outcomes research and the implications of applying the results. The goal is to improve health and health care.

Models for Population Health Improvement by Health Care Systems and Partners: Tensions and Promise on the Path Upstream: Proceedings of a Workshop (2022) This report provided a summary of an extensive discussion about population health improvement and collaboration with healthcare systems and other partners focused on higher level of actions to improve health.

Vital Directions for Health and Health Care: Priorities for 2021 (2021): In 2021, the NAM reassessed the priorities and issues of urgent attention for the next administration and published several commentaries in *Health Affairs*.

- *Vital Directions for Health and Health Care: Priorities for 2021*
  This report identified the overarching theme of this series as the clear and urgent obligation for the United States to turn its full attention

to the growing problem of health inequities as well as structural racism, which perpetuates health disparities.

- *Infectious Disease Threats: A Rebound to Resilience*
  This report reviewed pandemic preparedness in the United States and outlined steps to strengthen the country's ability to anticipate and respond to future pandemics.
- *Optimizing Health and Well-Being for Women and Children*
  This report applied a life-course framework to identify promising interventions to improve the health of women and children.
- *Actualizing Better Health and Health Care for Older Adults*
  This report identified six strategies to improve care and quality of life for older adults.
- *Transforming Mental Health and Addiction Services*
  This report described new models of care that focus on mental health and addiction.
- *Healthcare Costs and Financing: Challenges and Strategies for a New Administration*
  This report discussed health costs and financing priorities to advance health care access, affordability, and equity.

Source: National Academy of Medicine. (2021). Vital directions for health and health care: Priorities for 2021. *Health Affairs.* https://www.healthaffairs.org/health-policy-priorities-2021

Examples of Other Reports

- *Collaboration Between Health Care and Public Health* (2015)
- *The Future of Home Healthcare* (2015)
- *Informed Consent and Health Literacy* (2015)
- *Health Literacy: Past, Present, and Future* (2015)
- *Community-Based Health Literacy Interventions* (2018)
- *Improving Access to and Equity of Care for People With Serious Illness* (2019)
- *School Success: An Opportunity for Population Health* (2019)
- *A Roadmap to Reducing Childhood Poverty* (2019)
- *Virtual Clinical Trials: Challenges and Opportunities* (2019)
- *Integrating Social Care Into the Delivery of Health Care: Moving Upstream to Improve the Nation's Health* (2019)
- *Population Health in Rural America in 2020* (2021)
- *Faith Health Collaboration to Improve Community and Population Health* (2021)

- *Evolving Crisis Standards of Care and Ongoing Lessons from COVID-19* (2022)
- *Improving the CDC Quarantine Station Network's Response to Emerging Threats* (2022)

Access to IOM/NAM Reports

The NAM publishes many reports annually. The reports and other IOM/NAM resources can be read online or downloaded for free using the guest status. Full or parts of reports can be reviewed. There is no fee to access these reports. This information can be accessed at https://nam.edu/publications/.

References

Finkelman, A. (2017). *Teaching the IOM: Implications of the IOM Reports for Nursing Education, Vol. I* (4th ed.). American Nurses Association.

Finkelman, A. (2017). *Learning IOM, Vol. 2* (4th ed.). American Nurses Association.

QSEN Institute. (2020). *QSEN Institute competencies.* https://qsen.org/competencies/

Index

D

E

F

G

H

About the Author

Anita Finkelman, MSN, RN is a nurse educator and consultant, currently providing services in the U.S. and Israel, where she has been visiting faculty at Recanati School for Community Health Professions at Ben-Gurion University of the Negev and consulted with several Israeli universities. She served on the nursing faculty at Bouvé College of Health Sciences, School of Nursing, Northeastern University, where she taught undergraduate and graduate online courses and led the nursing school's CCNE accreditation process for undergraduate and graduate programs with full accreditation received. She previously served as an assistant professor of nursing at the University of Oklahoma College of Nursing, where she taught undergraduate and graduate nursing online courses and served as course coordinator for undergraduate nursing research. At the University of Cincinnati, Finkelman was an associate professor of clinical nursing, the director of continuing education, and the director of the undergraduate program (BSN), and taught public/community health, mental health nursing, nursing leadership, health policy, research courses, and clinical practicum. She has worked with several smaller colleges to develop and implement online programs and develop curriculum for pre-licensure nursing students.

Finkelman earned her BSN from Texas Christian University and her master's degree in psychiatric-mental health nursing/clinical nurse specialist from Yale University. She completed post-master's graduate work in healthcare policy and administration at George Washington University and participated as a fellow in the Health Policy Institute at George Mason University. Her nursing experience includes clinical, educational, and administrative positions and considerable experience developing distance education programs and curriculum, as well as a long history of teaching online. Finkelman has extensive management experience serving in various positions in psychiatric-mental health settings (acute care and community), having served as the director of staff education for two acute care hospitals and within clinical nurse specialist positions. As a consultant, she focuses on areas of curriculum and quality improvement, teaching-learning practices, distance education, healthcare administration and policy, nursing education accreditation, and assisting nurses in their publishing endeavors.

She has authored many books, chapters, and journal articles, served on journal editorial boards, and made presentations on nursing education, healthcare administration, health policy, healthcare quality improvement, continuing education, and psychiatric-mental health nursing, both nationally and internationally. She serves as a consultant to publishers in the areas of distance education and product development.

Finkelman's textbooks include *Professional Nursing Concepts* (Jones and Bartlett Learning, 5th ed., 2021); *Quality Improvement: A Guide for Integration in Nursing*, (Jones & Bartlett Learning, 2nd ed., 2020); *Leadership and Management for Nurses: Core Competencies for Quality Care* (Pearson Education, Inc., 4th ed., 2020); and *Case Management for Nurses* (Pearson Education, Inc., 2010). She has also authored chapters in M. Nies and M. McEwen's (Eds.) *Community Health Nursing: Promoting the Health of Aggregates*, Philadelphia, PA: W.B. Saunders Company.